10 Powerful Ideas for Improving Patient Care

Your board, staff, or clients may also benefit from this book's insight. For more information on quantity discounts, contact the Health Administration Press Marketing Manager at (312) 424-9470.

Library of Congress Cataloging-in-Publication Data

Reinertsen, James, 1947–
  10 powerful ideas for improving patient care / James L. Reinertsen and Wim Schellekens.
    p. ; cm.
  Includes bibliographical references.
  ISBN 1-56793-236-3 (alk. paper)
    1. Medical care—Quality control. 2. Outcome assessment (Medical care) I. Title: Ten powerful ideas for improving patient care. II. Schellekens, W. M. L. C. M. (Wim M. L. C. M.) III. Title.
    [DNLM: 1. Quality Assurance, Health Care—methods. 2. Quality Assurance, Health Care—organization & administration. W 84.1. R367z 2004]
  RA399.A1R456 2004
  362.1'0685—dc22

                                                                        2004059913

The paper used in this publication meets the minimum requirements of American National Standard for Information Sciences—Permanence of Paper for Printed Library Materials, ANSI Z39.48-1984. ⊗ ™

Acquisitions editor: Audrey Kaufman; Project manager: Jane C. Williams; Layout editor: Amanda J. Karvelaitis; Cover design: Trisha Lartz

Health Administration Press
A division of the Foundation of the
   American College of Healthcare Executives
1 North Franklin Street, Suite 1700
Chicago, IL 60606–4425
(312) 424–2800

Institute for Healthcare Improvement
20 University Road, 7th Floor
Cambridge, MA 02138
(617) 301-4800

Introduction

The work of healthcare leaders is changing. Hospital executives have traditionally viewed their primary responsibility as the stewards of the principal assets of the enterprise—investing capital in facilities and technologies and protecting the financial strength to continue those investments. The quality of clinical care, on the other hand, has commonly been viewed as the primary responsibility of practicing physicians and other clinicians, with the professional healthcare administrators (whether their background is clinical or not) playing a supportive, but not necessarily a leading, role.

The publication of *To Err Is Human* (Kohn, Corrigan, and Donaldson 2000) and *Crossing the Quality Chasm* (Corrigan, Donaldson, and Kohn 2001) has brought the clinical quality role of healthcare administrators to the foreground. The reports made clear to the public and to various regulators and payers that it is not enough that

hospitals are ensuring that their doctors have the proper credentials and are provided with good facilities and technologies. As a result of these findings, hospitals are feeling growing pressure from accreditation agencies and other regulators, as well as from new pay-for-performance initiatives, to produce the quality results the public deserves. This pressure falls squarely on the shoulders of healthcare administrators. In essence, it is causing healthcare leaders to reframe their view of their own work—from "I am responsible for healthcare facilities and assets" to "I am responsible for managing a clinical care delivery system."

Mary Pittman, chief executive officer (CEO) of the American Hospital Association's Health Research and Educational Trust, made this point very clearly at a 2004 meeting of hospital leaders. Her organization regularly surveys hospital CEOs to find out what is on their minds. For years, the list of CEOs who have said, "Clinical quality performance is my most important challenge" has been about a quarter of a page long. In the past year or so, however, this list has jumped to six pages—a striking change. As one CEO at the meeting stated, "I'm not surprised. There used to be four ways for hospital executives to lose their jobs: lose money, anger the doctors, fight with key board members, or get the hospital's name in the paper for something bad. Now there's a fifth: miss your clinical quality goals" (Reinertsen, Finucane, and Wallace 2004).

LEARNING HOW TO DO THE NEW JOB

How will healthcare administrators meet this new challenge? At a project level, for example, how will they lead teams to move from tepid, incremental results to dramatically improved performance? At an institutional level, how will they achieve the scale and spread necessary to be able to promise reliable, measurable, high-quality system-level results?

This book does not provide the answers to all of these questions, but it does meet one of a leader's most critical needs—a set of powerful ideas that addresses these types of leadership challenges.

To improve anything, leaders must develop the will to improve, generate strong ideas for improvement, and execute those ideas to bring about needed changes. This leadership model, first articulated by Nolan (2000) and subsequently expanded by the Institute for Healthcare Improvement (Reinertsen et al. 2003), is depicted in Figure A. This book focuses on the "Generate Ideas" part of the model.

WHY THESE IDEAS?

Hundreds of ideas come across the desks of busy healthcare executives and managers. How would they decide which ones might be useful to them in their work? We faced exactly this question when selecting the ten ideas to highlight in this book.

In our work around the world with quality improvement, we encounter many good ideas. To winnow these ideas down to the ten most useful, we used two tests.

First, the idea had to have caught and held our attention. Both of us are former CEOs of major hospitals and healthcare systems. We now function in facilitative and coaching roles for hundreds of leaders in healthcare organizations. As we considered each idea, we asked ourselves the following:

Figure A. Institute for Healthcare Improvement Leadership Model

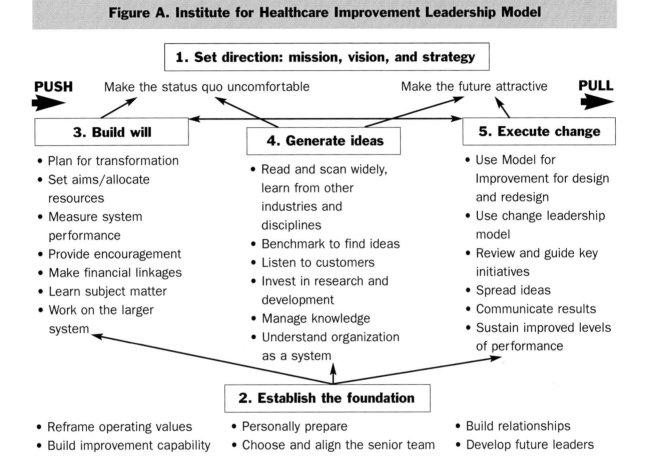

1. Set direction: mission, vision, and strategy

PUSH — Make the status quo uncomfortable — Make the future attractive — **PULL**

3. Build will
- Plan for transformation
- Set aims/allocate resources
- Measure system performance
- Provide encouragement
- Make financial linkages
- Learn subject matter
- Work on the larger system

4. Generate ideas
- Read and scan widely, learn from other industries and disciplines
- Benchmark to find ideas
- Listen to customers
- Invest in research and development
- Manage knowledge
- Understand organization as a system

5. Execute change
- Use Model for Improvement for design and redesign
- Use change leadership model
- Review and guide key initiatives
- Spread ideas
- Communicate results
- Sustain improved levels of performance

2. Establish the foundation

- Reframe operating values
- Build improvement capability
- Personally prepare
- Choose and align the senior team
- Build relationships
- Develop future leaders

Source: Institute for Healthcare Improvement, Cambridge, Massachusetts.

■ Would we want to use this in our own organizations?

■ Does this have appeal to leaders at multiple levels in an organization, not just to the CEO?

■ Does this have appeal across multiple clinical and other professional disciplines?

■ Is this being used?

The choices we have made are therefore intended to be useful to individual leaders at multiple levels of an organization and across clinical disciplines.

The second test was harder. Of each idea we asked, "Is this producing real results?" The answer to this question was an important consideration in narrowing the list down to ten, because ultimately results are the only measure of the value of an idea. Interestingly, results are also the ultimate measure of leadership (Drucker 1996).

We make no attempt to state that the chapters that follow discuss either the ten *best* or the ten *newest* ideas for improvement. Many of these ideas *are* new and therefore need to be disseminated more widely. A few of them have been around for a while but need to be reemphasized, in our view, if leaders are to achieve real results. We did not poll the quality improvement world to see what they believed the best ideas are. The list in this book simply represents the judgment of two seasoned executives about the ideas that have the broadest relevance to and highest impact on the quality challenges faced by today's healthcare leaders.

USING THIS BOOK

Each chapter of this book is devoted to one idea. First, the idea is described, and one or more specific examples of how that idea is being used are given along with some of the results observed. In most instances, we summarize why we think the idea is important and give suggestions on where the reader could turn to learn more about it. In some instances, there are bonus ideas within the chapter.

Many good ideas cluster together or nest within one another. For example, the "Move a Big Dot" idea applies mainly to executives who work at the organizational level. If the "big dot" that you choose to move, however, is the patient mortality rate, a number of practical ideas (e.g., the 2 x 2 Mortality Table) are given that are useful to those of you who work at the departmental or project level, such as a manager in the intensive care unit. Therefore, more than ten ideas are actually presented here.

This book may be used in several ways. First, simply read it right through—without any particular issue, project, or initiative in mind—as a review of what you already have in your portfolio of ideas and as a way of expanding that portfolio. Our hunch is that doing so may cause you to rethink some of the current approaches you have toward clinical quality, because one or more of these concepts will infect you just as it did us.

Second, scan the book for one or more ideas that would be directly applicable to a quality problem you are now facing. For example, if you are the executive within whose sphere of responsibility a bogged-down project falls, but you are not the actual project leader, you should be conducting regular executive reviews with the project team. One of your tasks as an executive is to diagnose whether the team's difficulties are due to lack of will, weak ideas, poor execution, or some combination of these issues. If "weak ideas" is your diagnosis, you and the team may look over this book to see if one or more of the concepts presented may jump-start better performance.

Third, read the book out of sequence. While all the chapters intersect in one way or another, they were designed to be understandable on their own, encouraging you to follow whatever sequence interests you.

Finally, the only way to really know an idea is to use it, or perhaps to teach it. We strongly suggest that leaders try out these ideas—in projects, organizational change initiatives, leadership-development curricula, and other activities necessary to improving clinical care. To paraphrase the German poet Goethe, knowing these ten ideas is not enough; we must apply them.

REFERENCES

Corrigan, J. M., M. S. Donaldson, and L. T. Kohn (eds.). 2001. *Crossing the Quality Chasm: A New Health System for the 21st Century*. Washington, DC: Institute of Medicine, National Academies Press.

Drucker, P. F. 1996. "Not Enough Generals Were Killed." In *The Leader of the Future*, edited by F. Hesselbein, M. Goldsmith, and R. Beckhard, xi-xv. San Francisco: Jossey-Bass.

Kohn, L. T., J. M. Corrigan, and M. S. Donaldson (eds.). 2000. *To Err Is Human: Building a Safer Healthcare System*. Washington, DC: Institute of Medicine, National Academies Press.

Nolan, T. 2000. "A Primer on Leading Improvement in Healthcare." Presented at the Fifth European Forum on Quality Improvement in Health Care, Amsterdam, March 24.

Reinertsen, J. L., M. Bisognano, L. Provost, T. Nolan, and W. Rupp. 2003. "Leading to Perfection: A Model of Leadership for Transformation." White paper. Boston: Institute for Healthcare Improvement.

Reinertsen, J. L., M. Finucane, and R. Wallace. 2004. "Straight Talk About Clinical Quality with Healthcare CEOs." White paper. [Online information on Ernst & Young web site; retrieved 9/20/04.] http://www.ey.com/us/healthsciences.

Put the Patient in the Room

Put the patient in the room—on every board, committee, task force, improvement project, and design group in your organization.

Healthcare leaders should see to it that patients are full participants on all improvement teams, board committees, cross-disciplinary task forces, and other groups that work on improving patient care. In other words, put activated, articulate patients (and family members) in the rooms in which decisions are being made about the design of their care processes and systems.

Put the patient in the room is not about focus groups or other similar methods by which healthcare leaders ask patients to react to improved care designs that doctors, ▶

nurses, and administrators have created. Neither is the idea about including patient preferences during the actual delivery of care, such as the setting of goals in a plan for chronic disease. Both of these are important practices, but they are not the primary focus of this idea.

Rather, this idea is about including patients in the process of redesigning care systems and bringing their input, concerns, and values into the improvement process from the beginning. The underlying belief here is that results will be better if patients are involved. It lies within the core principles of the Institute of Medicine's blueprint for a transformed healthcare system as outlined in *Crossing the Quality Chasm* (Corrigan, Donaldson, and Kohn 2001).

This method is an open and direct way of sharing control—shifting some power, if you will, from us to our patients and their families. As such, it raises a number of questions such as, "Whose room is it, anyway?" and "Why do we state the idea in such a controlling, paternalistic way?" If one way of framing the overall practice of patient-centeredness is to consider ourselves to be guests in our patients' lives, rather than patients to be guests in our organizations, should

the idea be rephrased to something like "put ourselves in our *patients'* rooms?" In other words, should we instead think of ourselves as guests on our patients' design teams, rather than the other way around? (Garrett 2004).

These are provocative questions, and they surface important tensions that need to be addressed. Let's see the ideas in action first, and return to the tensions later. Following are examples of how putting the patient in the room works in practice.

EXAMPLE: SHARED CARE PLAN AT ST. JOSEPH

St. Joseph PeaceHealth, a 250-bed hospital in Whatcom County, Washington, is leading a communitywide effort to redesign chronic disease care (see http:// www.ihi.org/IHI/Programs /pursuingperfection/). The leadership board for this effort includes all the members you would expect: CEOs; medical directors; and executives from various clinics, physician practices, and health plans. It also includes someone you would not expect: Rebecca Bryson, an informed, activated, articulate patient with several chronic diseases, including diabetes and congestive heart failure.

Ms. Bryson is cared for by 11 physicians in 5 different organizational settings, and she is on an average of 10 medications. When one physician changes a medication dose, or stops one to start another prescription, Ms. Bryson informs the other 10 physicians of her new drug regimen. (Otherwise, she has learned that she will suffer the consequences of adverse drug events and other problems.) Early on, she asked the healthcare administrators on the leadership board, "Why can't you do this for me, and for yourselves?"

This heartfelt, reasonable question broke through interorganizational rivalries that are common in communities like Whatcom County. It also allowed the leaders of otherwise independent entities to commit to the development of a communitywide, electronic Shared Care Plan for patients with chronic disease. Not surprisingly, a critical requirement of the plan specified by the leadership board was a common medication list, which is updated for all caregivers.

Ms. Bryson describes her role on the leadership board this way: "Patients can help to lead transformational change, even though we have no power or authority. We are the great levelers. When it comes to setting the direction or breaking through the ties, they all yield to me as if I were the boss. That's what becoming 'patient-centered' really means" (Bryson 2003).

The actual design process of the Shared Care Plan involved patients with chronic disease, which was critical to the outcome. As Dr. Marc Pierson (2003) states, "There is no way that information technology experts, physicians, and nurses would have come up with the designs that the patients wanted, if they hadn't been in the room with us."

An example of patient input is evident in the opening page of the Shared Care Plan record (see Figure B). This first page contains what patients believe is important for their care team to know, such as their personal long-term goals and the location of their advance directives. Normally, billing and demographic information opens any health record.

Results

With the Shared Care Plan at the core, and a number of other patient-centered designs in its chronic care system, hundreds of St. Joseph PeaceHealth's diabetics are starting to see real results. Nearly 50 percent of these patients now have glycosylated hemoglobin levels less than 7 percent.

Figure B. Shared Care Plan Record

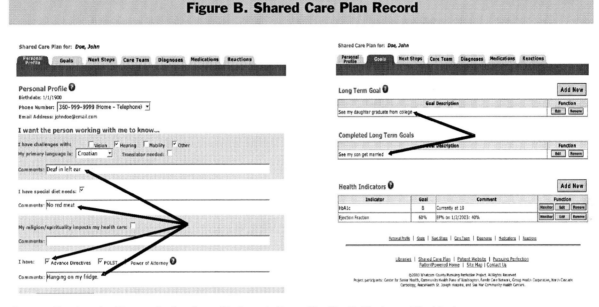

Source: Reprinted with permission from St. Joseph PeaceHealth, Bellingham, Washington.

EXAMPLE: PULMONARY REHABILITATION AT KING'S COLLEGE

The Pursuing Perfection team at King's College Hospital in London, England, set itself the challenge of improving care for patients with chronic obstructive pulmonary disease (COPD). One of the team's major obstacles was to redesign the system of pulmonary rehabilitation, which had long wait times, high costs, and low patient satisfaction levels. A key strategy in the redesign effort was to enlist patients with COPD in the design process from the outset. COPD patients were not only delighted to participate, they also came up with a number of significant "breakthrough" ideas.

For example, the COPD patients noted that each patient was unique in level of knowledge, desire for self-management, severity of disease, and other characteristics. With the guidance of the patient-run Breathe Easy group, the rehabilitation team redesigned its service from a one-size-fits-all eight-week course to a menu of education and rehabilitation options tailored to the needs and wishes of individual patients. Patients with high self-management skills and mild disease now can choose a much more streamlined, lower-cost program, whereas more dependent, severely ill patients receive the intense, full 12-week course (see Table 1).

Results

Twice as many COPD patients now start the process of rehabilitation, and three times as many complete the entire process. Wait times are down, as are the overall costs of the rehabilitation service. Most importantly, the early going shows a nice improvement in level of pulmonary function for this COPD population. Almost half the patients have moved to a higher level of self-management and/or pulmonary function.

WHY IS THIS IDEA FIRST ON OUR LIST?

1. *It is a powerful driver of cooperation*. Organizations have learned that when patients are sitting at the same table as doctors, nurses, pharmacists, and CEOs, their presence tends to stifle self-serving and organization- or profession-centric discussions.

2. *The presence of patients brings the whole system of care out into the open*. They experience care across multiple departments, physician offices, and institutions. Their presence on design teams opens the eyes of those responsible for those systems to new ways in which cooperation can drive improvement. Ms. Bryson's question about communitywide medication lists ("Why can't you do this for me?") rings constantly in the ears of the physicians and administrators who have heard it. After a few meetings with patients like Ms. Bryson present, many administrative leaders simply cannot go back to viewing their responsibilities as separate from the larger community care system. And that's a good thing.

3. *Patients have innovative ideas that get results*. The designs and outcomes of the Shared Care Plan for Whatcom County and the pulmonary rehabilitation system in South London would never have been as successful if patients had not stopped the designers and said, "No, that's not going to work for us. Why don't we try it *this* way?"

4. *The experience of being part of these committees helps patients to understand the science of medicine and the strengths of the care system as well as its weaknesses*. Patients who are so informed can serve an enormously useful "linking" role to other patients and the broader community, educating and

Table 1. Designing Pulmonary Rehabilitation to Fit Patients' Characteristics

	Mild Disease	Medium Severity	High Severity
High Self-Management	• Leisure card • Smoking cessation • COPD booklet/disk • Breathe Easy • Cost: $120	• Leisure card • Exercise on referral/walks • Self-help management course • Smoking cessation • Cost: $300	• 4/52 pulmonary rehab in leisure center • Exercise on referral/walks • Self-help management course • COPD booklet/disk • Referred to buddy patient • Cost: $460
Medium Self-Management	• Leisure card • Exercise on referral/walks • Self-help management course • Smoking cessation • COPD booklet/disk • Breathe Easy • Cost: $300	• Leisure card • Exercise on referral/walks • Self-help management course • Smoking cessation • Referred to buddy patient • Cost: $450	• 7/52 pulmonary rehab in leisure center • Breathe Easy • Smoking cessation • Crisis management • COPD booklet/disk • Referred to buddy patient • Cost: $650
Low Self-Management	• 4/52 pulmonary rehab in leisure center • Exercise on referral/walks • Breathe Easy • Self-help management course • Smoking cessation • COPD booklet/disk • Referred to buddy patient • Cost: $580	• 7/52 pulmonary rehab in leisure center • Exercise on referral/walks • Breathe Easy • Smoking cessation • COPD booklet/disk • Referred to buddy patient • Cost: $580	• 7/52 pulmonary rehab in hospital • PLUS 4/52 in leisure center • Breathe Easy • Smoking cessation • Crisis management • COPD booklet/disk • Referred to buddy patient • Cost: $880

Source: Reprinted with permission from King's College Hospital, London, England.

informing them about what's really going on.

5. *Physicians and nurses have found that patients on design teams bring an enormous reservoir of emotional support for healthcare professionals.* Patients want those who care for them to feel good about their work, and they will do everything in their power to ensure the success of the professionals to whom they are entrusting their lives.

If you are a CEO looking for a radical transformational strategy for your organization—one that will drive fundamental, deep changes in your culture, organizational design, core processes of care, and relationships with the rest of the community—we can think of no idea stronger than this: put the patient in the room—on every board, committee, task force, improvement project, and design group in your organization.

AVOID THE PITFALLS OF THIS IDEA

Put the patient in the room is strong medicine and can backfire if you do not use it well. Among the early lessons are as follows:

1. Be as thoughtful about which patients you choose to put on boards, task forces, and design teams, as you would about which administrators, physicians, and nurses you put on those design and decision-making groups. People, including patients, are not equally gifted in their ability to see beyond the boundaries of their own experiences; to speak articulately for the needs of others; or to bring a positive, can-do attitude to the group.

2. Patients (and parents, in the case of pediatrics) tend to have more good improvement ideas, and more long-term engagement on design teams, when the design problem revolves around chronic illness rather than around an acute problem or one-time diagnostic service.

3. No doubt that this idea raises some potentially awkward power and control issues for professionals and for patients. In practice, however, patients' ideas about how to design care (e.g., Ms. Bryson's request for a system that would keep track of chronic disease patients' medication lists) are seldom wacky or scientifically unsound. Although there are times when "doctor knows best" and a patient's suggestion needs to be trumped by medical science, those occasions appear to be far less frequent than expected. In other words, we can consider ourselves "guests on our patients'

design teams" without sacrificing the science of medicine.

4. It seems prudent to place several patients on any design team, rather than to count on a single patient's voice to bring the full range of ideas and concerns forward, especially in such a potentially intimidating environment.

One last note: be prepared for consequences, because once you start down this road, there is no going back. As Dennis Malloy, COPD patient and chair of the Lambeth Breathe Easy group in South London says, "You've given us the lollipop, and we're not giving it back."

WHERE TO LEARN MORE

There are a number of resources to which you might turn, over and above the chapters on patient-centeredness in *Crossing the Quality Chasm*. If you wish to see truly innovative work being done in patient-centered information systems design for chronic disease, go to www.patientpowered.org. This web site describes the Shared Care Plan as it continues to develop in Whatcom County.

For anyone wishing to understand an overall framework for engaging activated patients, an important resource is the web site www.improvingchroniccare.org. It is devoted to sharing the chronic disease model first articulated by Wagner and colleagues (2001).

An entire section is dedicated to chronic disease on the superb web site www.ihi.org. This section is full of good ideas on and approaches to putting the patient in the room.

REFERENCES

Bryson, R. 2003. Interview with author, March 24.

Corrigan, J. M., M. S. Donaldson, and L. T. Kohn (eds.). 2001. *Crossing the Quality Chasm: A New Health System for the 21st Century*. Washington, DC: Institute of Medicine, National Academies Press.

Garrett, S. 2004. Interview with author, April 6.

Pierson, M. 2003. Interview with author, March 3.

Wagner, E. H., R. E. Glasgow, C. Davis, A. E. Bonomi, L. Provost, D. McCulloch, P. Carver, and C. Sixta. 2001. "Quality Improvement in Chronic Illness Care: A Collaborative Approach." *Joint Commission Journal on Quality Improvement* 27 (2): 63-80.

Move a Big Dot

Big dots are system-level measures of performance.

The history of quality improvement in healthcare largely revolves around projects, for which a department, patient care unit, or individual office practice forms a team, applies improvement science, makes changes, and shows a measured enhancement in one or more quality attribute. An innovation group at the Institute for Healthcare Improvement has come to call these project-level improvements the *small dots*, perhaps because they are usually accompanied by plot-the-dots run charts with which teams display performance data over time. These are in contrast to the *big dots*, which are system-level measures of performance. ▸

There is nothing intrinsically wrong with project-level improvement. In fact, capable project work lies at the core of quality. Far too often, however, healthcare projects fade away because they require continued special effort and resources and are not woven into the fabric of everyday operations of any hospital or clinic. An even more common shortcoming of the project approach is that it fails to spread and scale throughout the organization. The result is that while the projects provide opportunities to learn about quality improvement, recognize staff, and generate CEO photo-ops for the hospital annual report, they usually do not noticeably change the performance of the whole system.

The problem is summed up in the following statement (Reinertsen, Finucane, and Wallace 2004):

> In other words, the history of quality improvement looks as if we had spent 15 years proving, in project-level work, that we could land various types of boats carrying different kinds of soldiers and equipment onto different parts of the coast of France, but we had never learned how to mount a full scale attack—to invade Normandy—to achieve and sustain system-level quality results across many conditions, simultaneously.

THE BIG DOTS

Big dots are system-level measures of important things that patients notice in a hospital, healthcare system, or physician group practice. Examples are the following measures proposed by an innovation group at the Institute for Healthcare Improvement (IHI), charged with developing practical, system-level measures of performance that correspond to five of the six quality dimensions forwarded by the Institute of Medicine—effectiveness, efficiency, safety, patient-centeredness, timeliness, and equity. (A detailed measurement kit is available—see Nelson et al. 2004.)

1. Safety: Adverse drug events per 1,000 doses
2. Safety: Workdays lost per 100 employees per year
3. Effectiveness: Hospital standardized mortality rate
4. Effectiveness: Functional outcomes for specific major conditions
5. Patient-centeredness: Patient satisfaction
6. Patient-centeredness: Percentage of patients dying in hospital within the region

7. Timeliness: Days to third next-available office or clinic appointment
8. Efficiency: Healthcare costs per capita for region
9. Efficiency: Hospital-specific standardized reimbursements

This list is obviously just a starting point. A growing number of healthcare leaders in the United States and Europe are beginning to use these and other system-level measures as a way to guide their strategies for improvement. Their organizations are also committed to sharing their results with each other to drive faster learning and establish a sense of urgency and public accountability for improvement. In contrast to relying on the project-by-project approach, these organizations and their leaders are taking aim at the big dots. They are focusing on the whole quilt, not on the individual patches.

EXAMPLE: THE HOSPITAL STANDARDIZED MORTALITY RATE

All of the measures listed above are important system-level performance attributes, but one in particular seems to stand out from the rest: "alive or dead after the hospital experience," or more formally, the *hospital standardized mortality rate (HSMR)*. In contrast to many other measurements, death is an unambiguous, all-or-nothing event that is recorded with high reliability. The mortality database, therefore, is more accurate than those for other quality measures.

Furthermore, everyone is in agreement about what "better" is when it comes to mortality rates. Patients, families, physicians, nurses, regulators, and politicians all want to avoid needless deaths.

Sir Brian Jarman has provided a very helpful, highly adjusted measure of hospital mortality rates by applying his years of work on British hospitals to the U.S. Medicare database (Jarman, Nolan, and Resar 2003). This particular big dot has provided some useful early learning about how leaders approach the challenge of moving an entire system to better performance.

Perhaps the most important lesson from the early work on HSMR is that when leaders work from the big dots in, they come up with a fundamentally different improvement agenda than when they work from the project level out.

For example, consider the following question: If your hospital successfully completes two projects in evidence-based medicine—one for acute myocardial infarction and the other for hip replacements—will those projects tend to move your mortality rates in the right direction? Almost everyone would answer the question with, "of course." As a result, healthcare leaders have historically sent out assignments to their managers and physician leaders, such as "everyone should work on two evidence-based improvement projects this year." This approach may allow the hospital to pass the quality improvement requirements of the Joint Commission on Accreditation of Healthcare Organizations, but it is not a plan to move a big dot.

On the other hand, leaders whose primary aim is to make a substantial improvement in a big dot such as HSMR face a different question: "What combination of initiatives (projects) will be powerful enough to reduce our hospital's mortality rate by 30 percent?" The quality improvement agenda that arises from answering this question is fundamentally deeper and more systemic than "everyone do two quality projects."

The plan to move a big dot may well include some of the projects that would be in the two-projects approach. The answer to this question, however, would constitute a quantitatively rigorous, integrated theory of a strategy to achieve a major change in a system-level performance measure.

Case of Tallahassee Memorial

The experience of Tallahassee Memorial Hospital in Florida is instructive. When its CEO Duncan Moore learned that Tallahassee Memorial's HSMR was 30 percent higher than the national average, he declared a new quality aim: to improve HSMR by 30 percent in the first stage, benchmark levels of performance in the second stage, and thereafter reach for perfection—no needless deaths. His successor Mark O'Bryant and the leadership team at Tallahassee Memorial have continued to take on this extraordinary challenge and are making real headway in reducing needless deaths.

Tallahassee Memorial's first task was to understand their patterns of death. In any hospital, some deaths are expected. Many hospital admissions are for purposes of providing comfort care only, and the outcome (death) is not only expected but even welcomed. For most admissions, however, the patients and the professionals who render care neither want nor expect death to be the result.

How would Tallahassee Memorial learn which types of patients were dying in the hospital, and where? They could not develop a plan of action until they understood the nature of the problem within their own institution.

(!) BONUS IDEA: 2 x 2 MORTALITY TABLE

When one takes aim at a big dot like a hospital's mortality rate, the aim often seems huge and formless. Tom Nolan has proposed a very useful idea for approaching hospital deaths, and this idea is applicable to many big, complex, system-level goals: stratify the problem into meaningful segments. Nolan's suggestion for hospital mortality is described as the 2 x 2 Mortality Table.

To create such a table, pull the charts of the last 50 consecutive deaths in your hospital and, using straightforward operational definitions (Jarman, Nolan, and Resar 2003), place each death into one of four boxes in the 2 x 2 table.

- Box 1: Patients admitted for comfort care only and to the intensive care unit (ICU) as the first stop in the hospital (i.e., patients admitted who were fully

2 x 2 Mortality Table		
	Admitted to ICU	**Not Admitted to ICU**
Admitted for Comfort Care Only	Box 1 **3.0%** (Range 0–14%)	Box 2 **13.3%** (Range 0–40%)
Not a Comfort-Care Admission	Box 3 **40.6%** (Range 16–64%)	Box 4 **43.2%** (Range 18–64%)

expected to die but who were placed in an ICU bed on admission)
- Box 2: Patients admitted for comfort care only and to a regular floor as the first stop in the hospital
- Box 3: Critically ill patients who were *not* admitted with comfort care only as the reason for admission (i.e., neither the hospital nor the patient intended that the patient should die) and who were admitted to an ICU as the first stop
- Box 4: Patients who were admitted to the hospital for some other reason than comfort care, who were not thought sick enough to put into an ICU as the first stop, and whose condition deteriorated during the admission and later died.

When the 2 x 2 Mortality Table was applied to the most recent 50 deaths in 27 hospitals, including Tallahassee Memorial, the results were as follows.

Boxes 1 and 2 do not contain needless deaths. They *do* represent interesting opportunities to improve end-of-life care planning and services in a community and to reduce unnecessary consumption of scarce resources such as ICU beds.

Box 3, on the other hand, contains many needless deaths, such as those of critically ill patients who develop ventilator-associated pneumonias (VAPs) or central line-associated bloodstream infections (CLABs), which "tipped them over." While these complications from critical care have been thought of as inevitable, they are not. A number of hospitals have essentially eliminated VAPs and CLABs; therefore, deaths caused by these complications have now become needless.

Needless deaths are also common in Box 4. The most common patterns of death in Box 4 (e.g., failure to respond to concerns of nurses about the deteriorating condition of a patient and failure of multiple physicians to develop and coordinate a plan of care) are extraordinarily important indicators of the cultural and organizational characteristics that determine reliability and resilience of

any given hospital. Box 4 is also where adverse drug events, thinly staffed nursing services, and other systemic hospital problems tend to show up.

After understanding its overall patterns of death, Tallahassee Memorial carefully reviewed charts in each of the boxes, especially in boxes 3 and 4. In Box 3, leaders found considerable opportunity to reduce VAPs, eliminate CLABs, and improve other aspects of critical care. In Box 4, they discovered that they shared a common pattern of death with many hospitals, particularly the pattern characterized by the label "failure to bring resources to the bedside of a deteriorating patient in response to a nurse's concerns."

With a clear understanding of its own patterns of death, Tallahassee Memorial's team has begun work on a broad and deep agenda. In their ICUs (Box 3), they are redesigning how critical care is organized and staffed and learning how to deliver evidence-based care with a high degree of reliability. On the non-ICU units, they are learning how to organize teams of experts who can come to the bedside of a deteriorating patient *before* the patient has a cardiac arrest and a Code Blue is called (at which point, of course, all the resources of the hospital are called to the bedside). The results are starting to come in (see Figure C).

Perhaps one of the reasons that quality improvement has not moved many big dots is that leaders simply have not aimed at moving them and therefore have not organized the work accordingly. We have tended to assume that if we moved lots of little dots through quality projects (e.g., if we applied evidence-based guidelines to several common diseases), then somehow all that improvement would move overall performance of the big

dots in the right direction. This practice has not proven to be true, however.

When a big dot like hospital mortality rate is studied, we find that the principal driver of "alive or dead after the hospital experience" is not whether evidence-based medicine is being used in every patient; instead, the drivers are system-level attributes such as nurse-physician teamwork, physician-to-physician communication, nurse staffing levels, end-of-life care planning in the community, and the staffing and organization of the ICU.

Figure C. Tallahassee Memorial Overall Mortality Rate

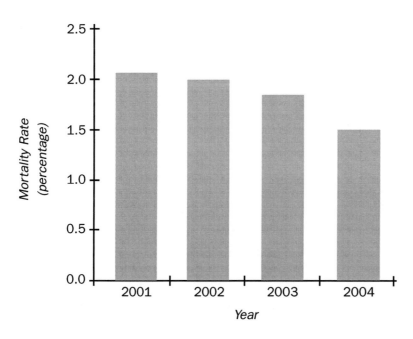

Source: Reprinted with permission from Tallahassee Memorial Hospital, Tallahassee, Florida.

WHY IS THIS IDEA IMPORTANT?

Tallahassee Memorial's work is early, as is the work of many organizations trying to improve their mortality rates. Their initial efforts, however, illustrate what happens to the quality agenda, and to the work of the management team and frontline staff, when an organization aims to move system-level performance measures. Among the lessons are the following:

1. *Moving a big dot requires that senior leaders declare the aim and make their commitment visible to their patients, governing board, and staff.* You will not achieve a fundamental change in system-level performance by keeping your intention to do so a secret.
2. *Your board must adopt the goal of achieving a new level of system performance.* The board must oversee, whether that goal is being achieved, with the same degree of rigor with which it oversees financial goals.
3. *You must channel executive attention to the aim.* Your personal schedule, meeting agendas, scheduled project reviews, and other methods of channeling attention must reflect the seriousness of this system-level goal.
4. *You must make achievement of the big dot a line-management responsibility.* This responsibility cannot be delegated to the quality staff, while the chief operating officer and unit managers work on other tasks.
5. *You must connect the movement of the big dot to your overall organizational strategic, operational, and financial plans.* In other words, the quality aim cannot exist in splendid isolation from the core work of the organization.
6. *You must drive scale and spread to achieve system-level change.* Your line managers will be looking for opportunities to spread improvements from one unit to another if they are accountable for moving a big dot.
7. *You must engage practicing physicians, or perhaps they must engage you.* Physician leadership and support are vital to many of the cultural and process changes (e.g., standardized practices) that are necessary to move big dots.
8. *Your choice of quality projects must change.* No longer should it be acceptable to ask every manager to work on two quality problems in

hopes that by the end of the year each manager's work will mesh into a significant improvement in system-level performance on important items such as adverse drug event rates, surgical wound infection rates, and overall mortality.

WHERE TO LEARN MORE

The best way to learn about moving a big dot is to get into action. The outline is simple, although the execution is not:

1. Take aim at moving a big dot, and link this quality aim in meaningful ways to your overall strategic plan. What will achieving this goal mean for your financial performance?

Market share? Regulatory compliance risks?

2. Select a measure—preferably one that you can track monthly—that will provide system-level feedback on whether you are moving toward your aim.

3. Form a theory of a strategy—the projects and other actions that will have enough depth and breadth to move the dot.

4. Implement the strategy, modifying it as needed based on the monthly feedback from your system-level measurement.

If you want to read a more comprehensive approach to system-level change than what is found in Jarman, Nolan, and Resar (2003), see Kaplan and Norton (1996).

REFERENCES

Jarman, B., T. Nolan, and R. Resar. 2003. "Move Your Dot: Measuring, Evaluating, and Reducing Hospital Mortality Rates." [Online information; retrieved 9/20/04.] http://www.ihi.org/IHI /Products/WhitePapers/MoveYourDotMeasuringEvaluatingandReducingHospitalMortalityRates.htm.

Kaplan, R. S., and D. P. Norton. 1996. *The Balanced Scorecard: Translating Strategy into Action*. Boston: Harvard Business School Press.

Nelson, E., K. Nolan, T. Nolan, D. Long, and B. Jarman. 2004. IHI's Health System Measures Kit: Version 1.0. [Online information; retrieved 9/20/04.] http://www.ihi.org/IHI/Topics/Improvement /ImprovementMethods/Tools/HealthSystemMeasuresKitIHITool.htm.

Reinertsen, J. L., M. Finucane, and R. Wallace. 2004. "Straight Talk About Clinical Quality with Healthcare CEOs." White paper. [Online information on Ernst & Young web site; retrieved 9/20/04.] http://www.ey.com/us/healthsciences.

Pursue
Perfection

When setting aims for improvement, set them in reference to the theoretical ideal.

Pursue perfection is an idea applicable to almost every improvement opportunity, independent of whether the opportunity is clinical, administrative, project level, or organizational level. Here's the idea: When setting aims for improvement, set them in reference to the theoretical ideal.

For example, if you are working to reduce deep sternal wound infections in cardiac surgery and your current rate of these infections is 3 percent, how should you frame your aim if

- statistically significant improvement would be 2.2 percent,
- the best local competitor is at 1.5 percent, and
- the world benchmark is 0.6 percent? ▸

Zero is the theoretical ideal for deep sternal wound infections. Pursuing perfection does not accept any ultimate aim other than the theoretical limit. Think of it this way: How do you explain to your patients that you are targeting to achieve a certain number of infections, needless deaths, adverse drug events, or delayed appointments? How do you ask patients to volunteer to be among the 2 percent who get an infection, among the 4 percent who die from the procedure, among the 1 percent who experience a serious adverse drug event, or among the 30 percent who wait needlessly for care?

EXAMPLE: ACUTE MYOCARDIAL INFARCTION AT MCLEOD REGIONAL

McLeod Regional Medical Center is a large community hospital serving the PeeDee Region of South Carolina, and it is a participant in The Robert Wood Johnson Foundation's Pursuing Perfection program. McLeod's leaders chose to work on the reliable delivery of evidence-based care for acute myocardial infarction (AMI); it was one of the projects through which McLeod would learn what it really took to "pursue perfection."

McLeod's baseline performance was pretty good: its doctors, nurses, and pharmacists were delivering all six indicated evidence-based services for AMI patients about 80 percent of the time. The first question McLeod faced was, "What should we aim for?"

Rather than work toward the available benchmarks (about 90 percent) or at "statistically significant improvement" (depending on the number of patients treated, this is approximately a 5 to 7 percent improvement), McLeod set its target at the theoretical ideal and framed its aim as a promise to patients: 100 percent of AMI patients would receive all six indicated evidence-based services.

Aiming high (perfection) caused McLeod's leaders to think differently about the whole project. Conventional approaches to this problem (e.g., education, communication, and data feedback to medical staff; training for nurses and other professionals) were likely to produce conventional results and, at best, benchmark performance. If McLeod were to approach and sustain perfect performance, it would need to think and act differently.

For example, within two months of the initial intense campaign for perfect AMI care, McLeod briefly hit

100 percent and then promptly fell back into the high 80s. This is a common observation in healthcare improvement. A sort of "Hawthorne Effect" occurs initially, followed by a return to previous behavior patterns. If McLeod's aim had been modest, its leaders might have been satisfied. However, McLeod was going for perfection, so it took additional actions to drive performance toward 100 percent.

One such action was related to discharge instructions. Three medications—aspirin, ACE inhibitors, and beta-blockers—needed to be discussed 100 percent of the time in discharge instructions if McLeod were to hit its goal. Hospital leaders had tried to address this medication issue by putting in place an AMI-specific discharge instruction process, but despite this new process, 10 percent or more of patients still were not receiving the proper medication plan. Building on advanced concepts of high-reliability organizations, leaders realized that the problem was not that they had a defective process for delivering

Figure D. Compliance with Six Indicators of Care for AMI Patients

N=98	N=62	N=63	N=79	N=57	N=63	N=94	N=77	N=69	N=75	N=68	N=59	N=75	N=59
Jan-02	Feb-02	Mar-02	Apr-02	May-02	Jun-02	Jul-02	Aug-02	Sep-02	Oct-02	Nov-02	Dec-02	Jan-03	Feb-03

Source: Reprinted with permission from McLeod Regional Medical Center, Florence, South Carolina.

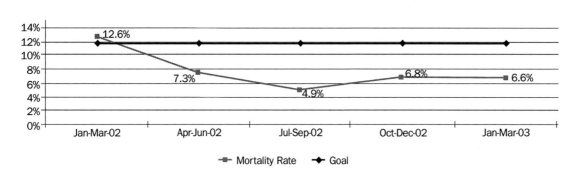

Figure E. Mortality Rate of Patients with Primary Diagnosis of AMI

Source: Reprinted with permission from McLeod Regional Medical Center, Florence, South Carolina.

evidence-based discharge instructions for AMI patients. The issue was that the hospital's discharge process was unreliable for all patients!

Therefore, McLeod implemented a systemwide discharge process that not only brought its evidence-based AMI care up to 98 percent to 99 percent but also improved the discharge communication and planning for all patients (see Figure D on page 25).

Most importantly, this quality project was not just an exercise in following guidelines for their own sake. McLeod's improvement in delivery of evidence-based care has been associated with a substantial decrease in the death rate of its AMI patients, from average to near-benchmark levels (see Figure E).

WHY IS THIS IDEA IMPORTANT?

Setting aims at the level of the theoretical limit has several important effects:

1. *It drives innovation*. You cannot achieve breakthrough performance with conventional ideas or with minor tweaking of current processes.
2. *It removes complacency*. Aiming to be a little bit better implies that current performance is not all that bad. Current performance, however, is not acceptable in many respects; see, for example, the RAND report showing that only 55 percent of needed evidence-based services are delivered to chronic

disease patients (McGlynn et al. 2003). Aiming high puts current performance in stark relief.

3. *It centers on what patients care about.* None of our patients want defective care. They certainly would not be satisfied with benchmark performance if they knew that benchmarks contain so many defects.

4. *It spurs deep systems change.* When you take something to 100 percent or zero, whichever perfect is, you usually must change aspects of your information management, routine work flow, human resources policies, and other systems that improve *all* your services, not just the specific problem you are trying to address.

(!) BONUS IDEA: TRY THE T ½ FORMULA

For those of you who are saying, "But these goals are unattainable— targeting perfection would discourage my staff," you might try Tom Nolan's related idea of the T ½ of improvement—that is, set an intermediate aim to close the gap between current performance and perfection by half. For example, you could first aim to reduce sternal infections from 3 percent to 1.5 percent (halfway to perfection) in six months. Once you reach that target, your next aim would be to take infections from 1.5 percent to 0.75 percent in the following six months, and so on, thereby asymptotically approaching perfection.

In case this is not obvious already: this idea is definitely *not* about benchmarking, for which Jim Buckman at the University of Minnesota's Juran Institute has a wonderful definition— "Benchmarking: a method for becoming the cream of the crap." In an industry that produces tens of thousands of needless deaths every year and where even the best institutions experience overuse, underuse, and misuse, we should aim higher than being the "cream of the crap." We should target the theoretical ideal.

WHERE TO LEARN MORE

Two collaborative quality improvement initiatives have placed the pursuit of perfection at the center of their efforts. The Pittsburgh Regional Healthcare Initiative, under the leadership of Paul O'Neill, is challenging all the providers in the Pittsburgh, Pennsylvania, region to aim at the theoretical ideal. The initiative's work in hospital-acquired infections, among other efforts, is gaining real traction. For example, West Penn Allegheny General Hospital has shown that CLABs can be essentially eliminated. Read more at www.prhi.org.

The Pursuing Perfection program, which is composed of 13 organizations/communities in the United States and Europe, has worked toward a goal of achieving the theoretical ideal for three years. The results of their efforts (such as McLeod's story and similar successes at Hackensack University Medical Center in New Jersey and Tallahassee Memorial in Florida) should inspire us all to aim at blowing right through the benchmarks. Many of the lessons from this experience have been distilled and brought forward online at www.ihi.org.

REFERENCE

McGlynn, E. A., S. M. Asch, J. Adams, J. Keesey, J. Hicks, A. DeCristofaro, and E. A. Kerr. 2003. "The Quality of Health Care Delivered to Adults in the United States." *New England Journal of Medicine* 348 (26): 2635-45.

Indicators Are the Cheese, Not the Whole Sandwich

It is wasteful and possibly dangerous to measure indicators without having both a purpose for doing so and an action plan for the outcomes.

When physicians are in training, they are taught over and over again not to order laboratory tests without a purpose and an action plan. Their mentors pepper them with questions such as, "What are you looking for in this test?" and "What will you do differently if the laboratory test shows an abnormal result?" Lab tests are expensive, sometimes even dangerous, so it is not a good idea for doctors to indulge their curiosity by ordering them thoughtlessly.

Administrators and regulators trying to improve healthcare may benefit from a similar lesson contained in this idea: *Indicators are the cheese, not the whole sandwich.* ▶

Health system leaders (and their boards) often become very interested in establishing overall indicators of performance such as balanced scorecards, minimal data sets for hospitals, and other measurement sets. These system indicators of performance can be much like physicians' lab tests—that is, it is wasteful and possibly dangerous to measure them without having both a purpose for doing so and an action plan for their outcomes.

The indicators, or measurements, are like slices of cheese. The purpose or aim and action plan act as the bread, without which you cannot make a quality improvement sandwich.

THE ROOTS OF THIS IDEA

This idea is grounded in the framework for all improvement—the three questions that must be asked as you begin the improvement process, as defined by the Model for Improvement by Langley and colleagues (1996):

1. What are we trying to accomplish? (the *aim* question)
2. How will we know that a change is an improvement? (the *measurement* or *indicators* question)

3. What change can we make that will result in improvement? (the *action plan* question)

Leaders who say, "Give me a good set of indicators for my organization so that I can report it to the board on a quarterly basis" without asking and answering the other two questions may make their boards happy but are unlikely to improve care.

EXAMPLE: FOUR-COLUMN TABLE AT BRADFORD TEACHING HOSPITALS

David Jackson is the CEO of Bradford Teaching Hospitals, a "three-star" or "most highly rated" acute care hospital in the British National Health Service. He has clearly articulated the aim for improvement of this care system: to become a place with no unnecessary deaths, no unnecessary pain, no feelings of helplessness for patients and staff, no delays, and no waste.

In addition to these transformational quality aims, Bradford also has aims that may be termed "staying-in-business requirements," such as access to capital and compliance with regulatory measures. Together, the transformational aims and staying-in-

Table 2. The Four-Column Table

Projects and Initiatives	System-Level Measures and Indicators	Staying-in-Business Requirements	Strategic and Transformational Aims
A description of the specific projects that in aggregate may move key system-level measures far enough in the right direction to achieve aims such as the following: • Use of evidence-based "bundles" in ICU care • Surgical wound infection reduction • ER flow management	• Mortality rate • ER wait time • Patient satisfaction • Staff turnover • Operating margin • Cost per case • Regulatory measures	• Access to capital • Growth • Regulatory compliance	No unnecessary • Deaths • Pain • Waits • Waste • Helplessness

Source: Reprinted with permission from Bradford Teaching Hospitals Trust, Bradford, England.

business requirements define the system-level measurements that will inform Jackson and other senior leaders whether Bradford is on course toward its goals. These system-level measures, in turn, can guide the selection and design of projects. Leaders can pose the question, "What combination of projects and other initiatives could move these system-level measures in the right direction?"

Visually, this work can be presented in a four-column table (see Table 2). The question, "What are we trying to accomplish?" is answered in the third and fourth columns. The question, "How will we know that a change is an improvement?" is addressed in the second column. The question, "What change can we make that will result in improvement?" is the topic of the first column.

Once completed, the table constitutes a theory of an organization's overall strategy for improvement. Generally, it is a good idea to work this four-column table from right to left.

At Bradford, two of the key indicators being monitored are mortality rate (see Figure F) and ER wait times (see Figure G). So far, Bradford's projects and initiatives in reducing wait times have produced stunning results, whereas efforts toward decreasing its mortality rate are still in the early stages. This may explain why the number of patient deaths has not yet fallen below the lower control limit (see Figure F).

Jackson knows, however, that if the mortality rate does not show improvement, then the activities in the first column will need to be modified. In other words, the measures in the second column are like a necessary lab test: Jackson knows why he ordered the measurement and has a plan for what to do when the measurement returns.

WHY IS THIS IDEA IMPORTANT?

Far too many organizational and regulatory leaders devote expensive resources to the development and production of indicators that are not tied to either an aim or an action

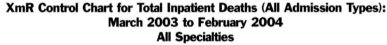

Figure F. Mortality Rate

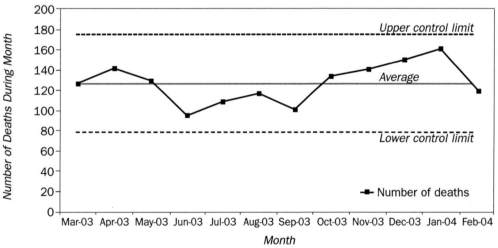

Source: Reprinted with permission from Bradford Teaching Hospitals Trust, Bradford, England.

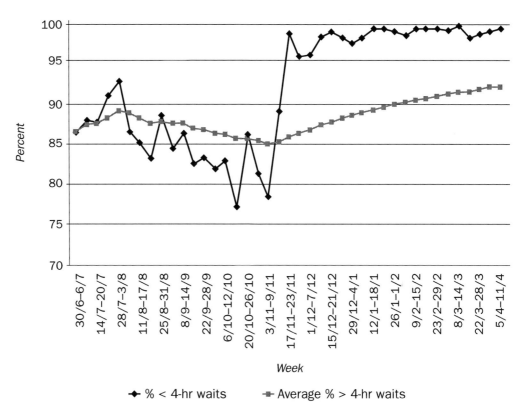

Figure G. ER Wait Times

% under-4-hour waits in Accident and Emergency by week versus average % of over-4-hour waits, June 2003 to April 2004

Source: Reprinted with permission from Bradford Teaching Hospitals Trust, Bradford, England.

plan. In our view, if you are the director for quality improvement or the vice president of medical affairs and your CEO asks you to "develop a balanced scorecard to present to the board on a quarterly basis," you are perfectly within your rights to ask two questions of your CEO:

1. What is our strategy and our aim so that I know what indicators of progress toward that aim I should put into the indicator set?
2. Supposing you had a set of reports on the following indicators, what would you do with them?

If these questions are not answered well, your organization will waste valuable time and energy on measurements that are not really important to its aims. Therefore, your organization runs the risk of becoming passive, rather than action oriented, about the measurements it does review, and it will miss major opportunities for improvement.

Ultimately, this idea is about preparing a whole sandwich, not just eating a slice of cheese.

REFERENCE

Langley, G. L., K. M. Nolan, C. L. Norman, L. P. Provost, and T. W. Nolan. 1996. *The Improvement Guide: A Practical Approach to Enhancing Organizational Performance.* San Francisco: Jossey-Bass.

Practice Science as Teams, Art as Individuals

If physicians practice the science of medicine as a professional team, society might give them the autonomy to practice the art of medicine.

All would-be leaders of improvement face a common challenge: engaging physicians to work *on* the system of care in addition to their critical role *in* the system of care. The idea described in this chapter engages physicians, getting them to examine and reframe one of their most cherished professional values: individual clinical autonomy. Here is the idea: *If physicians were to practice the science of medicine as a professional team, society might give them the autonomy they need to practice the art of medicine as individuals* (Reinertsen 2003). ▸

BUILDING THE TOWER OF BABEL

Consider what happens in a typical hospital immediately after grand rounds, in which a guest lecturer presents the latest evidence for caring for a particular condition. Some doctors change their practices immediately and put in place standing order sets and other reminders that embed the new evidence into their daily work. Others use the new information sporadically, or when they remember to do so. Others ignore the information entirely for a variety of reasons, ranging from skepticism to simple inertia.

In other words, there is enormous variation in how physicians in this theoretical hospital apply the evidence from the lecture. When this example is multiplied by hundreds of grand rounds and other ways of learning, by hundreds of conditions and across hundreds of doctors on the medical staff over many years, it becomes understandable that the orders that flow through the nursing and pharmacy departments in hospitals resemble the languages spoken at the Tower of Babel.

One result of this doctor-by-doctor approach of implementing evidence is the hundreds of physician-specific standing order sets in any given hospital. When hospitals tally their existing standing order sets, they typically find unique sets for each doctor, and it is not uncommon for a single physician to have several different orders of different vintages on the same condition (e.g., sliding-scale insulin). It is rare to find a hospital in which the medical staff has developed one set of sliding-scale insulin orders (or start heparin or pre-op preparation for bowel resection orders, for that matter) used hospitalwide by *all* physicians.

This problem is not restricted to inpatient practice. Even physicians who practice in groups seldom develop and use common approaches to common conditions, preferring to custom craft their treatment plans from scratch each time. Is it any wonder that only 55 percent of the evidence-based preventive and chronic disease services are delivered by the U.S. healthcare system (McGlynn et al. 2003)?

Culturally, physicians talk about evidence in groups but implement it as individuals. The resulting complexity and variation in orders is a breeding ground for errors and mishaps. When results suffer and patients are harmed, society acts to reduce physician autonomy through regulatory and health plan oversight of medical decisions. In a very interesting paradox for physicians, hanging on to clinical autonomy has become one of the causes of losing it.

ⓘ BONUS IDEA: STANDARDIZE CARE WITHIN, NOT JUST TO, THE EVIDENCE BASE

If physicians choose to practice science as a team, they face an interesting problem: the evidence base for many situations is ill defined; therefore, most of the hundreds of individual standing orders mentioned above can be argued to be evidence based.

If we allow variation to flourish within the broad evidence-based goal posts, we will continue to generate enormous complexity, mistakes, patient injuries, and wasted resources. This raises another idea, at least equal in importance to *practice science as a team*: standardize practices within, not just to, the evidence base. In other words, do not be satisfied just because each physician's version of care can be defended as being in accordance with the evidence-based standard of care. The variation that is permitted by such standards is far too broad.

Within a given hospital or clinic, physicians need to define and standardize their work within that broad evidence base, if breakthrough levels of quality and safety are to be achieved.

Example: Mediastinitis at Beth Israel Deaconess

Mediastinitis (organ space infection) is an extremely serious problem after cardiac surgery. Despite having rigorously standardized the procedures for preoperative antibiotics and the process of scrub, prep, and drape, the cardiac surgery and anesthesia team at Beth Israel Deaconess Medical Center in Boston was still experiencing a mediastinitis rate of 1.2 per 100 operations.

As a team, the surgeons reviewed the evidence for tight glucose control as a means of reducing infection and agreed that achieving such control (blood glucose levels targeted at 80 to 110) would be desirable. No set protocol existed, and there was controversy about how aggressively to administer insulin.

The team then agreed to "practice the science of medicine as a team." They all agreed to use one protocol and assess their results every six to eight weeks, making improvements to the protocol as indicated by how well glucose was controlled and by how many episodes of infection and hypoglycemia (a complication of insulin therapy) occurred.

Initially, insulin was administered only for patients with known diabetes and fairly high blood-sugar levels. By reviewing the results and making changes over time, the team learned to place all patients with glucose levels over 110 on the protocol, regardless of diabetes history. Blood-sugar levels were superbly controlled, without an increase in hypoglycemia. The most striking result of all is that it has been over a year since any episode of mediastinitis after cardiac surgery has occurred at the hospital.

Example: Evidence-based Bundles at Baptist DeSoto

Darla Belt, director of quality review for the 200-bed Baptist Memorial Hospital DeSoto in Southaven, Mississippi, has led a remarkable process of improvement in the institution's 28-bed ICU. The focus has been on *bundles* of services—sets of evidence-based practices that cluster in space and time and that should be delivered for every patient in a particular situation.

For example, strong evidence supports that every ventilated patient should receive the following bundle of services:

- Head of bed elevated 30 degrees
- Peptic ulcer disease (PUD) prophylaxis
- Deep-vein thrombosis (DVT) prophylaxis
- Mouth care every 2 hours
- Sedation vacation every 24 hours
- Aggressive weaning
- Insulin protocol to keep blood sugar under tight control (followed by some hospitals)

Note that these services (with the possible exception of the insulin protocol) are not really controversial and rest on a very solid evidence base. Furthermore, as Darla Belt (2004) says, "For some reason, bundles come across differently from protocols and care pathways. They make sense to physicians." Perhaps the reason for this is that these services seem like a natural evolution from other bundles that physicians have accepted for years, such as the sterile technique practices that every surgeon follows each time he or she scrubs for surgery.

How did Baptist DeSoto get the physicians on its open-staff ICUs to use the above-mentioned bundle for each ventilated patient every time? First, the ICU team instituted multidisciplinary rounds on every patient every day, reviewing the application of the ventilator bundle (and subsequently,

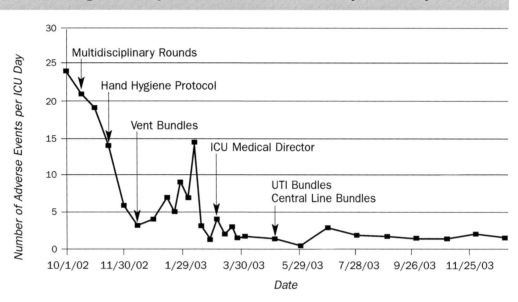

Figure H. Baptist DeSoto Adverse Events per ICU Day

Source: Reprinted with permission from Baptist Memorial Hospital DeSoto, Southaven, Mississippi.

for similar bundles focused on reducing central line-associated bloodstream infections and urinary catheter-associated infections). The team did not ask that the physicians standardize *how* they did PUD or DVT prophylaxis—at first. However, after a few months of getting used to the multidisciplinary team rounding on their patients and asking about the bundles, the physicians were ready to adopt a common set of protocols for these processes, and they did so because it made sense to them to have a common approach. The physicians also started to notice a dramatic effect on reducing adverse events such as ventilator-associated pneumonias and other complications of intensive care (see Figure H).

As more physicians learned of the significant impact of this simple change, the idea started to spread to other services and regular floors. Multidisciplinary rounding has been a key aspect of the spread of evidence-based practices. As one physician said of his experience having "his" patients rounded on by these expert teams, "It's as if you were having somebody important coming to visit your house. You like to have your house in order!"

The spectacular results have had another effect on the medical staff: they have become far less patient with the few colleagues who resist everything. At Baptist DeSoto, the medical staff are now the ones who ask those providers who refuse to use evidence-based bundles questions such as, "Are you so good that you are exempt from all the evidence in the literature?"

Interestingly, this story provides yet another example of how high quality costs less, not more. As Baptist DeSoto's nosocomial infection rates have plummeted, so have their costs per ICU stay (see Figure I).

How to Pursue the Bonus Idea

- The medical staff should undertake a systematic review of all current, standing order sets and initiate a sensible process for converting individual sets to sets used by all medical staff. This is particularly important when considering implementation of computerized order-entry systems. Computerized order entry will not improve safety much, if all that is being computerized is the unintelligible Tower of Babel.
- Periodically, individual physicians on the medical staff should be assigned to compare new medical evidence to existing order sets. Such physicians should lead a process for updating the order sets if necessary.
- If physicians persist in writing orders for suboptimal medications such as Demerol, the medical staff should approve a process whereby a physician's orders, if contrary to the evidence, can be automatically overridden. In other words, the patient would not get Demerol, even if the doctor ordered it (automatic substitution).
- In many clinical circumstances, sets of evidence-based practices that naturally cluster in space and time should be bundled together to produce a more reliable way to implement several practices simultaneously (see ventilator bundle example above).

WHY IS THIS IDEA IMPORTANT?

Physicians who overcome their professional attachment to clinical autonomy (at least so that they practice the science part of medical care as a team) will have a dramatic impact on reducing unnecessary complexity in their own work and the work of all those around them. This will also improve reliability and decrease costs.

Another very important benefit is the creation of "slack" for physicians

Figure I. Baptist DeSoto Nosocomial Infection Rates and Cost per ICU Episode

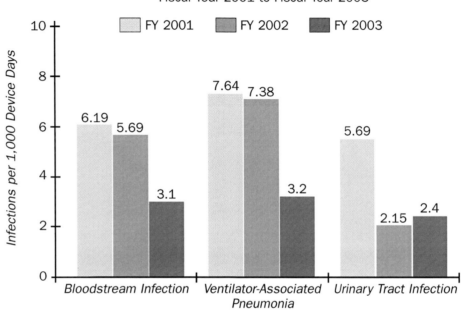

Nosocomial Infection Rates

Fiscal Year 2001 to Fiscal Year 2003

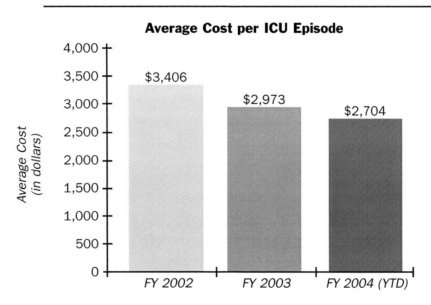

Average Cost per ICU Episode

Source: Reprinted with permission from Baptist Memorial Hospital DeSoto, Southaven, Mississippi.

and other professionals. Standardizing work within the evidence base gives physicians something they desperately seek: more time. It takes far less time to write "start heparin per protocol" than it does to write out the whole order set each time. What might doctors do with the extra time? There are three possibilities: see more patients, spend more time with each patient, or get home earlier.

This idea is a great way to engage physicians in the quality agenda.

WHERE TO LEARN MORE

As always, the best way to learn about this idea is to put it into action. On the inpatient side, see those teams who are working on prevention of surgical infections; ventilator-associated pneumonias; and other serious, well-defined harm events. The Institute for Healthcare Improvement's Breakthrough Series Collaboratives on ICU redesign and surgical infection provide a structured way to get experience at leading the implementation of this idea (see www.ihi.org/Programs /CollaborativeLearning).

In outpatient practice, preventive services seem to be an area where physicians can come to overall agreement fairly quickly and provide a good opportunity to learn what it means to implement a consensus, reliably, as a team.

A word of caution: it takes courage, knowledge of the evidence base, and confidence in your performance data to implement this idea well. As one superb leader of improvement stated, "When physicians insist on doing things their own way, contrary to the evidence, I simply say to them, 'so are you saying that you value your own autonomy more highly than the patient's outcome?'" (Isgett 2004).

REFERENCES

Belt, D. 2004. Interview with author, August.

Isgett, D. 2004. Presentation. Pursuing Perfection Milestone Meeting, Hackensack, New Jersey, April 28.

McGlynn, E. A., S. M. Asch, J. Adams, J. Keesey, J. Hicks, A. DeCristofaro, and E. A. Kerr. 2003. "The Quality of Health Care Delivered to Adults in the United States." *New England Journal of Medicine* 348 (26): 2635-45.

Reinertsen, J. L. 2003. "Zen and the Art of Physician Autonomy Maintenance." *Annals of Internal Medicine* 238: 992-95.

Adopt a Horizontal Process Orientation

Process orientation binds together all the specialties, departments, and organizations involved in providing optimal care to individual patients.

Patients often experience healthcare as a kind of archipelago—a collection of separate entities (or islands) that are made up of different disciplines, departments, and organizations; that do not communicate with each other; and that organize their care to suit their own interests, concerns, and budgets. Patients frequently get lost in this very complicated system, and more importantly they feel lost. They have no sense that anyone is responsible for the care pathway as a whole and that anyone is taking care of them as human beings. Island hopping is great for tourists in Greece, but it is devastating for patients who feel dependent and helpless. ▸

Patients need seamless care—a smooth flow from doctor to doctor, department to department, organization to organization—and care that is organized horizontally rather than vertically. We call this horizontal flow of care *process orientation*.

Process orientation binds together all the specialties, departments, and organizations involved in providing optimal care to individual patients, whether their illness is breast cancer, acute myocardial infarction, or diabetes mellitus (see Table 3).

A care process is a series of related diagnostic and therapeutic steps centered on a patient. Each step belongs to an "island" of a discipline, department, or organization; the process orientation of care binds these islands together for any group of patients.

The change of process orientation from vertical to horizontal requires a major shift in thinking and acting for most clinical staff (including doctors) and managers.

The results of a successful shift to process orientation include the following:

- The patient is central, rather than the doctor, department, or organization.
- New ways of collaboration focused on the patient develop across disciplines, functions, and organizations.

Table 3. Process Orientation of Care

	Outpatient Clinic	ER	Radiology	Lab	OR	ICU	Ward
Breast Cancer	Evaluation of new mass		Diagnostic mammogram		Mastectomy	Postoperative care	
AMI		Diagnosis		PTCA		CCU care	P-CCU care
Varices	Clinical diagnosis			Ultrasound	Vein stripping		Recovery
Diabetes	Diagnosis education			HbA1c			

Table 4. Vertical Versus Process Orientations of Care

	Vertical Orientation	Process Orientation
Grouping	Specialties, disciplines Departments Organizations	Care processes
Patient	Object of care	Subject of care
Focus	Doctors, managers	Patient groups
Efficiency Focus	Optimize the department	Optimize the overall care process
Collaboration	Around the doctors, within departments	Around the patient, crossing departmental borders
Nature of Care	Fragmented	Seamless
Leadership	United manager	Case manager, patient
Quality Emphasis	Doctors, departments	Patient

- Customer-supplier relationships are recognized among doctors, departments, and organizations.
- Care for patients is seamless, more effective, safer, more efficient, and more timely.
- The circumstances of work are more enjoyable and satisfactory for doctors, nurses, and other clinical staff as well as for managers.

The contrasting features of vertical and process orientations of care are summarized in Table 4.

VERTICAL ORIENTATION OF CARE

How does it happen that people who work in healthcare, whose primary purpose is to serve the needs of patients, focus so narrowly on their own specialty, department, or organization? Simply stated, this vertical orientation of care evolved historically because it is more convenient for clinical staff and managers and it is hard for everyone to "de-center" or shift from their own perspective to that of other people's.

Over time, these human tendencies toward self-orientation have been increasingly reinforced by powerful developments in the environment of medicine.

For many centuries, medical care involved a relatively simple relationship between a patient and a doctor, who was almost always a generalist. Several factors contributed to eliminating this simplicity, however. First, advances in knowledge and techniques created medical specialization. Today, there are over 30 different medical specialties, each of which takes care of ever-smaller parts of the human body and mind.

Second, medical technology has gone through enormous growth and continues to evolve. We now have x-rays, MRIs, PET scans, operating rooms, and different levels of care (i.e., home health care, intensive care, medium care, low care, day care, short-stay care, hospice care, acute care, urgent care, elective care, chronic care, and palliative care, each with its own special distinguishing characteristics). In some countries, family physicians or general practitioners function as gatekeepers who try, with variable success, to guide patients through the labyrinth that is healthcare.

Third, our hospitals have transformed from relatively simple to very complex institutions, with hundreds of doctors and residents and thousands of employees. Each hospital manages not only one core process, like an industrial company does, but at least 1,000 processes. In an attempt to make hospitals efficient, leaders built them around disciplines (e.g., surgery, internal medicine, obstetrics, pediatrics, dermatology) and departments (emergency room, radiology, endoscopy, operating room).

In a vertical organization, departmental managers are responsible for their own unit, and their concern is the production and budget within their assigned area of responsibility. The result is optimization of the departments and suboptimization for the hospital as a whole system.

In this environment, it is very difficult for the care providers to collaborate across boundaries. Who actually does care for the patient, especially at the transition points between the departments? How can the patient navigate in this "Balkanized" medical world?

Leaders' Role in the Problem

When I (Wim Schellekens) was CEO of an 800-bed, acute care teaching hospital, I noticed that patients in the clinical neurology department often stayed on that service for more than a week to wait for a CT scan, MRI, or some other test. Their care ground to a halt, as no other clinical decision could be made before the result of the test was reported.

I finally asked the manager of the radiology department why these patients had to wait that long. His answer was, "Each year you give me a fixed budget, and we make an agreement that I guarantee a certain quantity of production. Ninety-five percent of the patients come from outpatient departments, so it is very efficient to plan my production around those patients. Patients from the hospital services have to wait until I have a free slot for them. Every year you ask me if I've stayed within my budget and if I've reached my production target. This is the only way for me to make you happy."

In effect, the manager optimized the efficiency of his own department at the expense of the flow of inpatient care.

I realized that I was the problem! After all, what I asked my managers to do was run each of their departments as efficiently and productively as possible, rather than contribute to the overall care of patients and the results of the hospital as a whole.

Leaders' Role in the Solution

EXAMPLE: BREAST CARE AT REINIER DE GRAAF. The challenge to a breast service is straightforward: What is the best way to care for a woman who shows signs (e.g., a breast lump, an abnormal finding on a mammography screening) of breast cancer? To answer this question, leaders at the Reinier de Graaf Hospital in Delft, The Netherlands, did the following:

- Brought together all the disciplines and departments involved in the care of breast cancer patients, including surgeons; radiologists; pathologists; and staff from outpatient clinics, radiology, pathology, planning, and nursing. Together, they formed the improvement team. Their first task was to introduce themselves. For years, these people had worked together for this patient population, referring patients to each other and even complaining about each other's services, but they did not know one another personally nor had they even spoken to each other! This "bringing together" is one of the main tasks for leaders, as who else will take this initiative?

- Taught the basics of quality improvement to the improvement team, including setting aims, achieving balanced measurement, testing ideas in small cycles, and controlling and spreading the results.
- Asked the professionals to decide on the best way to manage these patients—that is, design an evidence-based, multidisciplinary protocol for diagnosis and treatment.
- Taught the group some change concepts from other industries, such as lean manufacturing, parallelization, pull instead of push systems, synchronization of processes around a specific time, segmentation of patient groups, and standardization of care.
- Encouraged the group to try out these change concepts in small cycles of testing (Plan-Do-Study-Act).

The results of this effort were remarkable:

- Access time was reduced to one day, rather than one week.
- Throughput time (cycle time) to reach a diagnosis decreased to half a day, instead of 10 to 14 days.
- Only one hospital visit was needed, rather than three.

- Only two surgeons, two radiologists, and three pathologists were involved, instead of a total of 21 caregivers.
- Two surgeons carried out the cytological puncture, rather than eight surgeons and eight radiologists.
- The puncture success rate increased from 60 to 95 percent.
- Patients were enormously grateful that they no longer had to wait 10 to 14 days to find out whether or not they had cancer. A woman who phoned for an appointment one day could have the results the following day by 12:30 p.m.
- The satisfaction of doctors and other workers was greatly increased; they enjoyed working this way.

EXAMPLE: STROKE CARE AT REINIER DE GRAAF. The same principles were used to redesign the care process of patients in the stroke service of the Reinier de Graaf Hospital, the Bieslandhof (nursing home), and the Sofiastichting (rehab center) in Delft, The Netherlands.

This care process is much more complicated because it involves not only different departments but also different organizations. The results of the process-oriented redesign were similarly successful (see Table 5).

Table 5. Results of a Process-Oriented Redesign

Attributes of Stroke Care in Delft	Baseline	After Process Redesign
Multidisciplinary, cross-organizational protocol	No	Yes
Collaboration: multidisciplinary, cross-departmental, cross-organizational	No	Yes
Mean length of stay in the hospital	28 days (5–195)	12 days (5–19)
Mean length of stay in the nursing home	100 days	60 days
Percentage of patients that returned to their home	30%	60%
Satisfaction of patients and families	Unknown	++++
Satisfaction of the caregivers	Unknown	+++
Financial results	High costs	Hospital: much less expensive Nursing home: more expensive Overall: less costs

The results of this project have now been spread to 23 regions in The Netherlands, using an approach similar to the IHI Breakthrough Series Collaboratives.

WHERE TO LEARN MORE

The following books provide more insight into the concepts presented in the chapter:

Juran, J. M. 1964. *Managerial Breakthrough: The Classic Book on Improving Management Performance.* New York: McGraw-Hill.

Langley, G. L., K. M. Nolan, C. L. Norman, L. P. Provost, and T. W. Nolan. 1996. *The Improvement Guide: A Practical Approach to Enhancing Organizational Performance.* San Francisco: Jossey-Bass.

Schellekens, W., and J. J. E. van Everdingen. 2001. *Kwaliteitsmanagement in de Gezondheidszorg.* (Dutch language). Houten, The Netherlands: Bohn Stafleu Van Loghum.

Walburg, J. A. 1997. *Integrale Kwaliteit in de Gezondheidszorg: van Inspecteren Naar Leren.* (Dutch language). Kluwer, The Netherlands: Deventer.

Walton, M. 1986. *The Deming Management Method.* New York: Putnam Publishing Group.

Use Statistical Process Control to Guide Dosage Adjustments

This idea can be applied in many healthcare processes unrelated to drug administration such as monitoring of blood pressures and heart rates.

Statistical process control (SPC) is hardly a new idea. When healthcare executives study quality improvement methods, one of the earliest lessons they learn is to "plot the dots"; that is, they learn to display the performance of a process graphically, over time, as a series of measurements. In its simplest form, plotting the dots results in the creation of a run chart, which provides a picture of both the degree of variation and any significant changes in the performance of a process over time. ▶

Fundamentally, a run chart provides a visual prediction of how the process will perform for the next patient or clinician who experiences the process. It is also a key method of answering the improvement question, "How would we know if the changes we made constitute an improvement?" (Benneyan, Lloyd, and Plsek 2003).

For example, consider the run chart in Figure J that displays a simple plot of the number of surgical site infections over time. An intervention (i.e., a change in the sterilization process for surgical instruments) was made at the time indicated. The visual impact of the data tells a very compelling story.

The ability to use and interpret run charts (and other more sophisticated SPC methods) has become an essential part of the management toolkit for any leader who wants to understand, predict, and improve the variation and performance of key administrative and clinical processes. A less-common use of SPC methods in healthcare is as an active management tool in "steering" any given process. The powerful idea for clinical quality and safety in this chapter is to *use statistical process control to guide dosage adjustments for high-hazard medications*.

As applied to medication management, the idea is pretty simple.

Figure J. Run Chart of Surgical Site Infections

Surgical Site Infections per Week

1. Understand the variation (by means of a run chart or control chart) in the current system of administration of Coumadin, anticonvulsants, antibiotics, or any other medication for which
   - a dose of medication is given for a period of time,
   - the medication blood level or some other lab test is checked, and
   - the dose of medication is adjusted in response to the blood level or lab test.
2. Each time a blood level or other lab test returns,
   - do not change the dose of medication if the test is within "common cause variation"—that is, do not respond to noise as if it were a signal;
   - if the lab test is outside the bounds of common cause variation (so-called "special cause"), investigate the situation and, if necessary, adjust the dose—that is, do not fail to respond to a real signal.

Basically, this approach uses SPC as a statistically solid way to separate a signal from noise in one of the most common daily events of any busy care delivery system's work—the administration of potentially hazardous medications (Wheeler 1999).

EXAMPLE: TACROLIMUS DOSING AT CINCINNATI CHILDREN'S

Tacrolimus is an immunosuppressive drug used in transplant patients. The drug has a narrow therapeutic range: give too little, and the transplanted organ may be rejected; give too much, and you damage the patient's kidneys or weaken his or her defenses against infection. The drug is powerful and potentially toxic. Moreover, it is given over months and years as a long-term method for controlling the immune response. While tacrolimus has substantially improved transplant graft survival, the medical literature advises physicians that 30 percent of patients who receive tacrolimus experience renal toxicity.

Cincinnati Children's Hospital Medical Center, a world-renowned transplant center, has always used the standard method for administering tacrolimus; that is, children would be started on a dose based on a guideline, blood levels of tacrolimus would then be measured at regular intervals, and physicians and nurses would adjust the dose according to the blood level. For example, if the tacrolimus level came back from the lab higher than the target range, the clinicians would reduce the dose a bit, based on their experience and judgment.

Figure K. Tacrolimus Levels in a Patient Over Time

Note: Target range is 4–9 ug/ml.

Source: Berwick, D. 2002. Plenary address at the Institute for Healthcare Improvement's National Forum, Orlando, Florida, December 5.

So how well does this process work? When the transplant team examined their performance on achieving target blood levels for tacrolimus, they were disappointed to find that this standard method of administering the drug produced tacrolimus levels in the desired therapeutic range only half the time. When the team plotted the dots for each child, they saw a picture of variation that was perhaps even more distressing—see Figure K.

With this finding, the team at Cincinnati Children's decided to apply SPC to the problem. They created run charts for each patient and established statistical "rules" for adjusting dosage.

These rules were based on SPC methods for determining whether any given blood level is just "noise" (i.e., the lab result represents normal variation and does not require any tacrolimus dose adjustment) or is a "signal" (i.e., the lab result is so different from the normal variation that it needs to be investigated and that a dosage adjustment may need to be made). In other words, the team decided to use statistical methods to make sure that they did not fiddle (or "tamper" in the SPC world; doing so makes variation worse) with doses when the lab results were just noise and that they did respond when the lab results represented real signals.

The new method produced much more predictable levels of tacrolimus. Consider the run chart in Figure L for the same patient after application of SPC to the management of her dose levels.

Don Berwick, president and CEO of the Institute for Healthcare Improvement, says the first rule of improvement is that "every system is perfectly designed to achieve the results it achieves." If that is true, the standard tacrolimus system of "check the lab test and make an individual judgment as to whether or not to change the dose" is perfectly designed to produce levels out of therapeutic range half the time and a high

frequency (up to 30 percent) of renal toxicity and other complications.

The new, nontampering system, on the other hand, is perfectly designed to produce a much lower risk of harm, while maintaining tacrolimus levels in the therapeutic range far more frequently.

Note that tacrolimus itself does not produce a 30 percent risk for renal toxicity, as stated in the medical literature. The way we administer tacrolimus creates the 30 percent risk; we have a propensity to tamper with medication dosages, which thereby increases rather than decreases variation in blood levels. Is this perhaps also true for many other

Figure L. Tacrolimus Levels in a Patient After Applying SPC

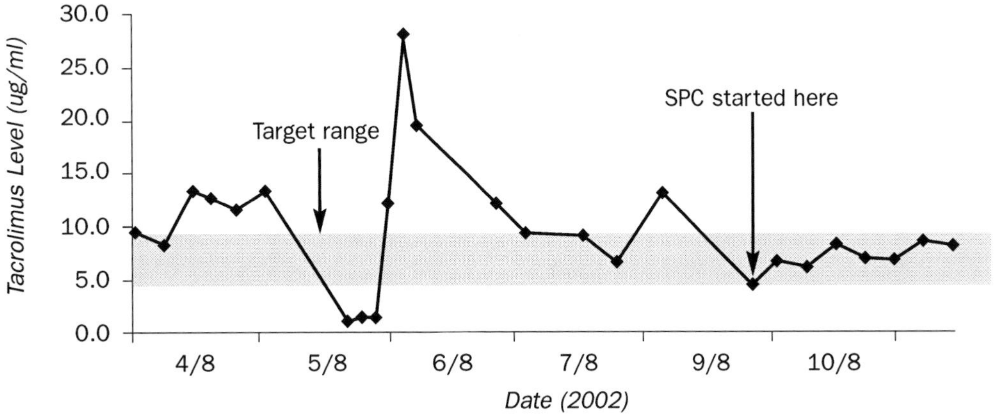

Source: Berwick, D. 2002. Plenary address at the Institute for Healthcare Improvement's National Forum, Orlando, Florida, December 5.

medications such as Coumadin, heparin, and anticonvulsants?

WHY IS THIS IDEA IMPORTANT?

Pharmaceuticals have become an extraordinarily effective part of our overall therapeutic capability. However, many drugs carry significant side effects, with anticoagulants, narcotics, immunosuppressives, and chemotherapeutic agents leading the list of medications associated with harmful events. The lesson from tacrolimus may well be that many toxicity problems with this and other drugs lie not with the drugs themselves but with the methods by which they are administered. In other words, while these medications have some dangerous properties, our methods of giving them are even more dangerous!

This idea can be applied in many healthcare processes unrelated to medication administration, such as monitoring of blood pressures, heart rates, and other critical indicators in the ICU. This idea is a good response to the Institute of Medicine's request in *Crossing the Quality Chasm*: "use the science we know." This is not simply an admonition to adopt evidence-based medicine practices; it is advising us to rely on all the improvement science we know (such as SPC) for our advantage.

WHERE TO LEARN MORE

There are many good texts on SPC. Donald Wheeler's *Understanding Variation: The Key to Managing Chaos, 2nd Edition* (SPC Press, 1999) is very accessible even if you are not a math whiz. For a broader, more comprehensive look at the subject, read *The Improvement Guide* by Langley and colleagues (Jossey-Bass, 1996). Carey and Lloyd's *Measuring Quality Improvement in Healthcare* (Quality Press, 2000) is a superb reference that includes many healthcare examples. It is particularly valuable for executives, managers, and clinical leaders who may not need to be technical experts in statistics but have to understand these principles to lead improvement.

REFERENCES

Benneyan, J. C., R. C. Lloyd, P. E. Plsek. 2003. "Statistical Process Control as a Tool for Research and Health Care Improvement." *Quality and Safety in Healthcare* 12 (6): 458-64.

Wheeler, D. 1999. *Understanding Variation: The Key to Managing Chores, 2nd edition*. Knoxville, TN: SPC Press.

Schedule
Discharges

The notion of making appointments for discharges arose to help hospitals deal with discharges and other flow-management challenges.

This idea is brilliant and relatively new: *make a specific discharge "appointment" for each inpatient.*

Discharges normally create an enormous burden for any inpatient unit. Generally, the signal to discharge the patient comes from a physician's order, which is written a few hours before the discharge is to take place. Following the receipt of this order, the nursing system, family members, and many other stakeholders begin a mad scramble to execute the order. ▶

To make matters worse, other patients on the same unit are usually going through the same process at the same time. Because most of this work happens between 10 a.m. and 3 p.m., it coincides with many of the admissions occurring on the same units, compounding the problem and causing a huge daily spike in the workload of nurses, housekeepers, social workers, and other key staff. When there is a back-up in discharges, other patients cannot be transferred from the emergency room and postsurgical recovery room to the regular floors. Essentially, delayed discharges are a critical bottleneck to the entire work flow of the hospital.

The notion of making appointments for discharges was conceived by Diane Jacobsen, Roger Resar, and Carol Haraden to help hospitals in an IHI Collaborative deal with discharge and other flow-management challenges. This idea originated from commercial aviation. When you fly from one city to another, your aircraft is allowed to take off (an admission to airspace) only when a slot is available for it to land at the destination (a discharge from airspace).

Hospital admissions and discharges do not normally work the way aviation does. We admit a patient to almost any open bed, even if the bed is not on a unit that cares for the specific illness of the patient. We also admit patients even when we do not have available beds, as we do not have a schedule for which beds will open soon. The resulting peak in work flow is one consequence. Errors, rework, and rushed communications with patients are other consequences.

This idea of scheduling discharges begins to address all of these problems, while helping to shorten length of stay in many instances.

HOW THE IDEA WORKS

First, create a certain number of daily appointment slots based on the number of patients that typically are discharged from the unit each day. For example, a typical unit may have a total of fifteen 30-minute discharge appointment slots available, starting at 9:30 a.m. and ending at 4 p.m.

Second, assign a specific discharge appointment slot to each patient as soon as possible in the care process. For patients who have undergone elective surgery, a discharge slot can usually be assigned even before admission (just like for commercial aviation). For other patients, a reasonable estimate such as "highly likely to be ready to go home in three days" can be made early in the admission. Once the care team has made such a prediction, they should give the patient an appointment for discharge in a specific slot—say, 11:30 a.m. on Thursday—at least 24 hours beforehand.

Third, and perhaps the most powerful step in this whole idea, post the date and time of the scheduled discharge appointment visibly in the patient's room and at the nurses' and physicians' work stations. Everyone who interacts with the patient—nurses, technicians, dietitians, social workers, family members, and house staff—can see the appointment and organize their work to match that discharge date and time. Knowing ahead of time gives them one to three days, rather than three hours, to complete the necessary tasks!

Having a discharge date can have a strong effect on patients' and families' outlook. Being in the hospital usually implies a serious illness, with many accompanying fears and uncertainties. Lack of a definite discharge date can unwittingly send a message to patients that their condition is bad—after all, if they were really getting better someone would have begun arranging for their discharge. To many patients and their families, knowing when they are scheduled

for discharge can be a tremendous relief.

On the other hand, some patients feel protected in the hospital, so having to face discharge can produce anxiety. Knowing several days in advance that their discharge is scheduled may stir up that anxiety, but it also gives the patient, family, and staff time to work through that feeling, which is something that cannot happen if the discharge is sprung on them on short notice. For all of these reasons, scheduling discharges is an important aspect of compassionate care.

When the discharge day and time arrive, the nurses' schedule is smoother and the work flow is evenly distributed throughout the day. This ensures that when a patient is being discharged at 11:30 a.m., five other patients are not being discharged at the same time.

EXAMPLE: DISCHARGE AT LEE MEMORIAL

Lee Memorial Hospital in Fort Myers, Florida, has taken a comprehensive approach to its flow-management challenges, and scheduling of discharges has been essential to its success. Lee Memorial has learned to use two different systems for predicting and scheduling patients' discharge appointments: surgical and medical.

For surgical patients, the prediction team consists of the surgeon, nursing team, patient, and family members. For medical patients, hospitalists work with the nurses and family to set a discharge appointment. After some learning, Lee Memorial now successfully discharges 80 percent of its patients within 30 minutes of the scheduled appointment time (see Figure M).

Once a reliable system of scheduled discharges from regular floors was in place, the staff at Lee Memorial could then match the transfer of patients from ICUs to a regular unit. Essentially, the ICUs know when beds will become available and can plan their transfers accordingly (see Figure N).

Efforts by staff at Lee Memorial have produced a significant improvement in the flow of patients from the emergency department into the rest of the hospital (see Figure O on page 62).

WHY IS THIS IDEA IMPORTANT?

1. *It directly addresses one of the most serious and disruptive*

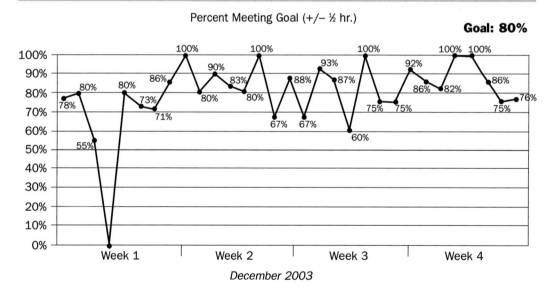

Figure M. Scheduled Discharges: Percent Occurring Within 30 Minutes of Appointment Time

Percent Meeting Goal (+/– ½ hr.)

Goal: 80%

December 2003

Source: Reprinted with permission from Lee Memorial Hospital, Fort Myers, Florida.

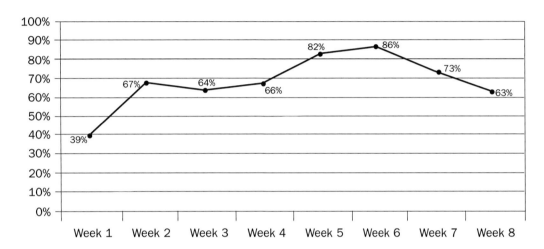

Figure N. Matching of Scheduled ICU Transfers to Scheduled Floor Discharges

MICU Scheduled Transfers
Weekly Average, 12/1/03 to 1/25/04

Goal: 80%

Source: Reprinted with permission from Lee Memorial Hospital, Fort Myers, Florida.

problems hospitals face—*flow management.*

2. *Nurses love it* because it gives them a sense of predictability and control over an otherwise unpredictable workday.

3. *It has enormous ramifications for the bottlenecks that can occur in many other upstream parts of the hospital,* such as operating rooms, emergency rooms, and ICUs. If staff have a good idea when and where beds are going to be available, they can plan their work flow accordingly.

4. *It improves patient satisfaction* dramatically because it drives a much higher level of communication and coordination among doctors, nurses, patients, and family members. It also has a powerful effect on patients' and families' expectations about recovery, which can be an important factor in overall outcomes.

5. *It is simple.* Implementation can be started next week.

6. *It works,* not just in acute care hospitals but also in nursing homes and other similar settings.

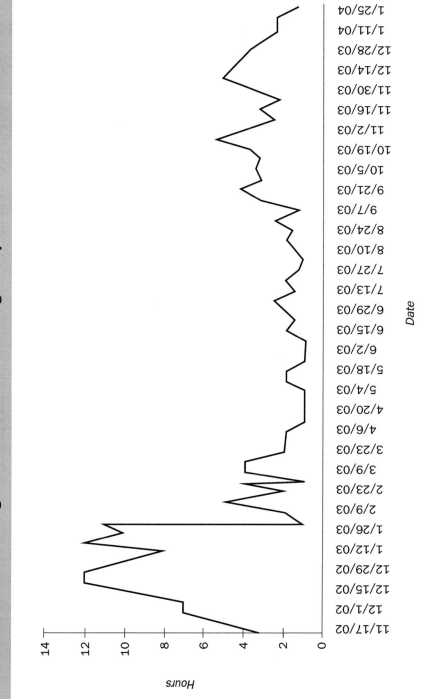

Figure O. Time from ED Discharge to Inpatient Bed

Hours

14 — 12 — 10 — 8 — 6 — 4 — 2 — 0

Date

11/17/02, 12/1/02, 12/15/02, 12/29/02, 1/12/03, 1/26/03, 2/9/03, 2/23/03, 3/9/03, 3/23/03, 4/6/03, 4/20/03, 5/4/03, 5/18/03, 6/2/03, 6/15/03, 6/29/03, 7/13/03, 7/27/03, 8/10/03, 8/24/03, 9/7/03, 9/21/03, 10/5/03, 10/19/03, 11/2/03, 11/16/03, 11/30/03, 12/14/03, 12/28/03, 1/11/04, 1/25/04

Source: Reprinted with permission from Lee Memorial Hospital, Fort Myers, Florida.

WHERE TO LEARN MORE

Scheduling discharge appointments is part of a larger flow-management system. The best way to learn more about the idea is to engage in the IHI IMPACT network initiative on flow management. A useful overview of this idea and of a more comprehensive approach to hospital flow can be found in the IHI white paper "Optimizing Patient Flow: Moving Patients Smoothly Through Acute Care Settings," which is available on www.ihi.org/IHI /Products/WhitePapers/Optimizing PatientFlowMovingPatientsSmoothly ThroughAcuteCareSettings.htm.

Implement the Nurse Capping Trust Policy

This approach not only addresses the capping question very effectively but also dramatically improves nurses' perception of control over their work environments.

The nurse capping trust policy is an organized system whereby frontline nurses—the ones doing the bedside work—are entrusted with answering the question, "Is it safe to admit another patient to this unit, given the patients we have, the number and skills of the staff on hand, the planned admissions and discharges to and from this unit today, and any other factors of which we are aware?"

Most hospitals have two systems of *capping*, or closing off new admissions to nursing units. ▶

The first is a formal system that involves complex negotiations between unit nurses and more senior nursing and administrative managers about workload, using data such as midnight census (which has almost no relationship to nursing workload, by the way). The second system is informal, by which nurses "cheat" to keep their units safe.

To understand the informal system, consider the following question, When a patient has just been discharged from a bed, and the nurses on that unit know they are swamped, do the nurses call housekeeping right away to clean the room so that a new admission can be put into that bed, or do they wait a few hours until things quiet down? About 30 percent of a hospital's potential capacity is blocked at any one time in the day through such informal methods of restricting access to beds.

The nurse capping trust policy takes a radical approach to this problem. Instead of leaders developing increasingly rigorous systems for measuring and controlling nurses' workload, and thereby allowing managers to make more precise decisions about when to cap nursing units, this idea entrusts the decision about whether to cap a unit to those who best understand the

safety issues posed by an additional admission to that unit—that is, the nurses on the unit itself.

This approach not only addresses the capping question very effectively but also dramatically improves nurses' perception of control over their work environments.

EXAMPLE: TRAFFIC LIGHTS AND HOSPITAL FLOW AT LUTHER MIDELFORT-MAYO

At Luther Midelfort-Mayo Health System in Eau Claire, Wisconsin, each unit's nurses decide their "workload tolerance" on a minute-to-minute basis. They use a traffic light system to communicate the unit's status to the rest of the hospital: red, orange, yellow, and green. Red means no admissions or capped, and the other colors denote progressively higher levels of workload tolerance (Rozich and Resar 2002).

To guide their decisions, the nurses developed a scoring method that takes into account key drivers of their workload, such as nurse staffing levels, number and complexity of patients, anticipated discharges and admissions, and nurse experience levels (see Table 6 for an example worksheet).

Table 6. Traffic Light Worksheet for a Cardiac Care Unit

Workload Tolerance Factor	Actual Status	Points
RN staffing	1:1 or less	0
	1.1 to 1.5:1	20
	1.5:1 to 2:1	30
	2:1 to 3:1	40
Tech staffing	14.1 or less	0
	None	10
Present census	11 or less	0
	12–13	10
	14	20
Anticipated turnovers	1–2	0
	3–5	10
	7–9	20
	10 or more	30
Staffing blocked beds	1	5
	2–3	10
	4	15
Discharge blocked beds	1–2	10
	3–4	20
	8	30

Total Points_____

Current status: Red_____   Orange_____   Yellow_____   Green_____

Would you like to change your status? Yes_____   No_____

Guidelines for points:

0 to 20: Green
20 to 39: Yellow
40 to 59: Orange
60 and above: Red

Source: Reprinted with permission from Luther Midelfort-Mayo Health System, Eau Claire, Wisconsin.

At any point in the day, as conditions change, unit nurses can revise the unit's status. If they decide the status is red, the unit's charge nurse coordinates that decision with the unit's medical director and then communicates it to the rest of the hospital in a variety of ways, including the traffic light system that functions as a screen saver on all the hospital's computers. The decision to cap a unit is made locally, without a need for senior nursing or other administrative review.

The decision to cap admissions is separate from determining whether or not the decision is appropriate. Appropriateness and frequency of capping are reviewed on a monthly basis, and corrections are made if necessary. The decision to cap a unit is never questioned in real time, however. In its three years of use at Luther Midelfort-Mayo, a decision to cap has never been reversed by more-senior administrators.

Results

Interestingly when nurses are given the authority to make the capping decision themselves, they do not abuse it. In fact, the frequency of capping of units at Luther Midelfort-Mayo decreased after this policy was put into place in February 2001 (see Figure P on page 68).

Not surprisingly, when the word of this policy got out into the nursing community (and this new policy was added to the rest of the hospital's recruitment efforts), nurse vacancy rates plummeted! In the five months following the implementation of the policy, the percentage of open positions in critical care units fell from 12 percent to 0 percent. Similarly, the overall hospital vacancy rate fell—from teen levels to low, single digits—during the year after the policy was initiated.

Hospital volumes, surgical admissions, and the percentage of time the hospital spent "on divert" because units (particularly ICUs) were capped could have been negatively affected by this policy, but for all of these measures, Luther Midelfort-Mayo has remained stable or has improved since implementation. Perhaps the strongest proof is that as of the summer of 2004, three-and-one-half years after its implementation, this policy is still a vigorously implemented feature of the overall system of patient-flow management at Luther Midelfort-Mayo. The nurse capping trust policy was not a 90-day wonder.

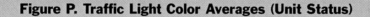

Figure P. Traffic Light Color Averages (Unit Status)

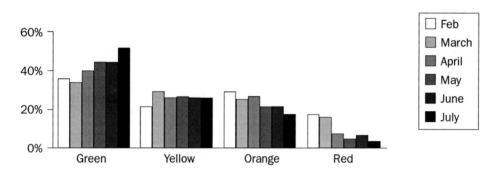

Source: Reprinted with permission from Luther Midelfort-Mayo Health System, Eau Claire, Wisconsin.

WHY IS THIS IDEA IMPORTANT?

At least three reasons make this a very powerful idea.

1. *It is a very effective way of dealing with one of the biggest headaches faced by nursing and hospital administrators—that is, making judgments about workload.* Most hospitals use administrative systems that try valiantly to come up with accurate methods using historical patterns, benchmarks, and real-time administrative data for deciding how to channel workload fairly, safely, and efficiently across diverse patient care units. The Luther Midelfort-Mayo example makes clear that

when it comes to patient safety, there is no substitute for the knowledge and judgment of the nurses doing the work themselves, particularly as they predict their work for the next few hours, which is something that administrative data systems do not seem to do well at all.

That nurses are capable of making judgments about workload should not come as a surprise. We trust nurses to make minute-to-minute judgments about the safety and medical care of patients; therefore, it is strange not to entrust them with decisions about their ability to accept an additional patient without jeopardizing the care of both the new and existing patients.

Incidentally, this idea also makes some hospital administrators and nursing leaders uncomfortable. A large part of their role as managers is ensuring that the nurse staffing budget is on target, as the single biggest expense category in the hospital budget is staffing. Therefore, managers are naturally threatened by an idea that asks them to give up control of this critical function (but not the accountability for hitting the staffing budget target). As one administrator, who preferred to go unnamed but seemed to speak for many others, phrased it: "It's akin to giving the keys to the asylum to the inmates."

2. *We like the "trust" part of the policy*, which has its roots in the wariness and distrust that goes both ways between administrators and line nurses, even when the administrators were former nurses themselves. Although the policy is not a magic bullet, it can repair a huge gap in the relationship between these two groups, which are two of the most important facets in any hospital culture. It is no accident that Luther Midelfort-Mayo named the idea the nurse capping *trust* policy.

3. *Perhaps the most powerful reason is that the policy has a positive effect on quality of care*, as would have been predicted by the work of Aiken and colleagues (2002) on nursing issues and quality. Aiken and colleagues have shown unequivocally that a very powerful predictor of quality and safety is the degree to which nurses perceive that they have control over their work environment.

We can think of no stronger method than letting nurses decide whether it is safe to take on another admission to reinforce their perception of control over the work environment. Frankly, given the workforce issues faced in nursing and the safety challenges faced by all hospitals, we do not understand why every institution has not rushed to implement the nurse capping trust policy.

REFERENCES

Aiken, L., S. Clarke, D. Sloane, J. Sochalski, and J. Silber. 2002. "Hospital Nurse Staffing and Patient Mortality, Nurse Burnout, and Job Dissatisfaction." *Journal of the American Medical Association* 288 (16): 1987-93.

Rozich, J. D., and R. K. Resar. 2002. "Using a Unit Assessment Tool to Optimize Patient Flow and Staffing in a Community Hospital." *Joint Commission Journal on Quality Improvement* 28 (1): 31-41.

Channel Attention to Improvement Projects

Attention is the currency of leadership.

Leadership can be thought of as "influencing people, processes, and structures to bring about needed change" (Reinertsen 2004). Leaders exert their influence and demonstrate their values and priorities through a variety of channels such as what they write and say and how they allocate resources.

Of all the resources that leaders allocate, time is what followers watch most closely; in particular, they pay attention to what leaders choose to do with their time. How a leader spends time or uses the "currency of leadership" is a significant determinant of what an organization works on and what it achieves. ▶

If attention is the currency of leadership, then leaders who wish to achieve significant quality improvements must channel it toward key leverage points for quality and must do so effectively.

IMPROVEMENT PROJECTS AND EXECUTIVE ATTENTION

Improvement projects are vital to the achievement of needed changes at the larger system level. If an organization does not deliver breakthroughs in projects at the unit or department level, it has nothing worth scaling and spreading to other parts of the organization. On the other hand, well-chosen projects—with high aims for improvement, capable project leadership and teamwork, and good organizational support—can raise the standard of care in the project area or department, promote spread throughout the organization, and demonstrate the values and behaviors that will ultimately drive systemwide quality transformation.

A project that produces real results—sustained improvement of a breadth and depth that makes both patients and caregivers notice—sends a signal to the entire organization that quality improvement is not just a sidebar activity. Conversely, a project that produces superficial results, is overpraised, or does not connect to overall organizational strategies also sends a signal that hinders, rather than accelerates, the achievement of systemwide performance improvement. For these reasons, projects are important leverage points—high-visibility moments in any organization's path to breakthrough performance.

Executive review of projects can influence whether the projects will succeed, scale, and spread. We have observed that as executives rise on the organizational chart, they often spend less of their personal time doing actual reviews with quality improvement teams, because more weighty responsibilities crowd project-level work out of their schedules. If the currency of leadership is indeed attention, and if leaders really wish to achieve major changes in quality performance indicators (such as mortality rate or the 39 indicators listed in the pay-for-performance project by the Centers for Medicare & Medicaid Services and Premier [CMS 2004]), then leaders, even senior executives, need to allocate at least some of their time to active, in-person, real-time engagement in key quality projects in their organizations.

Example: Bill Rupp, M.D.

Bill Rupp was the CEO of Luther Midelfort-Mayo for ten years. During his tenure, the system made a startling number of improvements such as making medical practice reliably evidence based, improving hospital flow management, and transforming the culture to one that values teamwork and process improvement as the core drivers of quality.

In an interview (Reinertsen 2004), Dr. Rupp discussed his role and how he used his personal time in the improvement process:

> I couldn't be personally responsible for guiding and directing specific projects like the traffic-light system, medication safety, and implementation of evidence-based care systems for specific diseases. But I could make sure the teams working on these problems knew that I was interested in them, and that I wanted results. I met monthly individually with the project leaders, even if only for 15 minutes, to hear about progress. And I also made sure that my executive assistant scheduled me to "drop in" for a few minutes on the meeting of each team at least once a month so that all the members of the team knew that the organization was paying attention to their work. I know this sort of attention must be important because when specific projects didn't go well (and we had a few), they were projects to which I didn't pay this sort of attention.

The first step is for executives to make the decision to channel attention to project reviews, and then budget the time in their own schedules for this activity. The next step is to learn how to do a good project review. It is not enough to give projects your time in a mechanical or perfunctory fashion. You must also know how to use that time well so that your reviews help, rather than hurt.

OUTLINE OF A SENIOR EXECUTIVE PROJECT REVIEW

Reinertsen, Pugh, and Nolan (2003) propose the following guidelines.

First, the purpose of reviews of projects by CEOs and other executives should be clear:

1. To learn whether the project is on track or is likely to fail
2. To understand why, if the project is not achieving the intended results
   a. Lack of organizational will
   b. Absence of strong enough ideas for improvement
   c. Failure to execute changes
3. To provide guidance, support, and stimulus to the project team on will, ideas, and execution
4. To decide whether the project should be stopped (too many executives complain that "nothing is ever allowed to fail in healthcare")

Second, good process review does not happen by walking into the team meeting and asking, "How's it going?" Maximum impact for your time comes from some premeeting preparation, a well-executed meeting process, and a system for postmeeting communication.

Here is a checklist for each step:

Premeeting Preparation

- *Know the context for the project.* Be prepared to remind the team why the project is important and how it fits into the overall goals and system-level measures of the organization. For example, if two key organization goals are reduction in mortality rates and decrease in costs per admission, and if the project being reviewed is aimed at improving inpatient flow, be ready to answer the question, "Why are we doing this flow project, and how does it relate to our strategic goals?"
- *Read the project report prior to the meeting.* A good general rule for reports is, "If even the CEO can understand the aims, measures, and results, it is a good report."
- *Communicate with the project leader to establish a meeting agenda and expectations.* A typical agenda would review aims, measures, results, prognosis, and ideas for next cycles of improvement. No "big" or very formal presentations are needed.

Meeting Process

- *Start the review by clarifying the aim.* Ask, "What exactly are you trying to accomplish in this project?" Look for aims set at the level of the theoretical ideal or that "raise the bar." Challenge more conservative goals.
- *Ask about the measurements.* Say, "Please summarize for me the measures you're using to know whether you're moving toward your aim." Look for a few solid

measures that are well defined and that have available comparative data.

- *Move to reviewing the results within three to five minutes of the review.* Look for graphic displays: graphs should be clear; sample size should be identified and preferably displayed as a time series. Spend considerable time on these results—enough time to establish that you understand the numbers, but more importantly that you really care about getting results.

- *Provide encouragement about some of the better aspects of the project.* Say, "Excellent use of stratification in breaking this project up into manageable chunks" or "You've already completed 16 improvement cycles? That's almost one every two days. Wow!"

- *Discuss trends and prognosis with the project team.* State, "Given your progress to date and the ideas you're planning to try, make a prediction. Are you going to achieve this project's aim?"

- *If there is any uncertainty about the project's prognosis, try to determine whether the failure mode is primarily related to will, ideas, or execution.* Indicators of each of these failure modes include the following:

Will:
—Resources necessary to the project's success are not made available
—A few loud naysayers are blocking implementation and spread of good ideas
—Obvious connection between this project and key strategic goals is absent
—There is lack of executive and board attention to this project
—Line managers appear to be on the sidelines and are not responsible for project success

Ideas:
—Project team has not gone outside the organization or outside healthcare to find the best ideas
—Few cycles of improvement have been attempted
—"Big ideas" appear to be absent; the changes being tested are safe and incremental, not radical redesigns
—Project team cannot tell you who has the best results in the world on this topic

Execution:
—Project setup and project management appear to be weak
—Preparation for spread is not part of the project from the inception
—Project team cannot articulate a coherent change-leadership

framework being used by the project

—Project gets good results on pilots but never seems to scale up

■ *If will seems to be the problem, the CEO or other senior executive often can make a major impact on changing it.* Make resources available, deal with the few loud voices, channel attention to the importance of this project, make the connections to key strategies, and/or assign responsibility to line managers.

■ *If ideas are the problem, ask questions such as the following that will stimulate the search for ideas:*

—What ideas do you have for further improvement?

—Where are you looking for new ideas? (Encourage the team to look far and wide, including outside of healthcare.)

—Who's the very best in the world at this? How can we find out? Give explicit permission and broad encouragement to try small-scale tests of big ideas. For example, say, "It sounds as if you have a number of good ideas already. How could you test one of those ideas and have an answer by the end of the week?" Senior executives doing a review have to be comfortable pushing

and supporting innovation and small tests.

■ *If execution is the problem, it is a good opportunity for you to teach good project management and change-leadership skills to the project team and to learn about the larger organization's barriers to execution in its culture, information systems, human resource policies, and other areas.*

■ *Conclude the meeting by describing what you have learned and understood about the project.* Also, ask, "Where do you need help from me?" Projects often encounter significant barriers within the organization, so it is important for the executive doing the review to understand how he or she can help the team reach its goals.

Postmeeting Follow-up

■ *Call or e-mail the team leader in a week, and periodically thereafter, to ask for the results of tests of change.* By doing so, your attention to the team will extend over a much longer time period, reinforce the importance of the team's work, and encourage many more cycles of improvement.

■ *Communicate to the team what you have done in response to members' requests for help.* This communication may be done at the next project review, but it may be more timely if it were simply an e-mail or other form of contact with team members.

COMMON FEARS AND ANTIDOTES

CEOs and other executives often avoid doing project reviews because of the following fears:

1. *They do not know much about clinical medicine or whatever the content of the project is.* The good news about the above checklist for doing a review is that executives can do reviews and do them well, without being content experts. It can even be an advantage to be a nonexpert because you can naively ask, "Why do you do it that way?," which sometimes causes major revisions in everyone's—even the experts'—thinking.

2. *They do not know the right quality language or how to interpret run charts and control charts.* "What if I ask a stupid question?" is a typical fear for senior executives. There are only two antidotes to this anxiety: knowledge (learn the basics of quality improvement so that you can ask meaningful questions about the results) and humility (do not be afraid to show your ignorance and to be taught by your team).

3. *They are concerned that such reviews are overstepping into a direct report's area of responsibility.* Obviously, you should not be doing the job of those who report to you, so assigning yourself to do every project review would be a legitimate concern. Is it not a good idea for senior executives to model good methods for doing reviews for the people who are directly responsible to them? This demonstrates what leaders want to emphasize and encourage.

REFERENCES

Centers for Medicare & Medicaid Services. 2004. "Rewarding Superior Quality Care: The Premier Hospital Quality Incentive Demonstration." [Online information; retrieved 11/20/04.] http://www.cms /hhs.gov/quality/hospital/PremierFactSheet.pdf.

Reinertsen, J. L., M. Pugh, and T. Nolan. 2003. "Executive Review of Improvement Projects: A Primer for CEOs and Other Senior Leaders." [Online information; retrieved 9/20/04.] http://www.ihi.org/IHI/Topics/Improvement/ImprovementMethods/Tools /ExecutiveReviewofProjectsIHI + Tool.htm.

Reinertsen, J. L. 2004. "Leadership for Quality." In *The Healthcare Quality Book: Vision, Strategy, and Tools*, edited by S. Ransom, M. Joshi, and D. Nash. Chicago: Health Administration Press.

ABOUT THE AUTHORS

JAMES L. REINERTSEN, M.D., is chief executive officer of The Reinertsen Group. Based in Alta, Wyoming, The Reinertsen Group is an independent consulting and teaching practice that helps healthcare leaders create organizational environments in which high-quality work by doctors and nurses can thrive.

In the past, Dr. Reinertsen has been an assistant clinical professor at the University of Minnesota in Minneapolis and a professor of medicine for Harvard Medical School in Boston. He was a subcommittee member for the Institute of Medicine's well-known reports *To Err Is Human* and *Crossing the Quality Chasm*. In addition, Dr. Reinertsen has written articles for major medical journals and is a nationally recognized speaker.

He is Senior Fellow at the Institute for Healthcare Improvement, where he heads the leadership development sector. He can be reached at jim@reinertsengroup.com.

WIM SCHELLEKENS, M.D., is the chief executive officer of the Dutch Institute for Healthcare Improvement CBO in Utrecht, The Netherlands. CBO is a not-for-profit knowledge center for innovation, implementation, and transfer of quality improvement models and instruments. CBO works closely with the Institute for Healthcare Improvement (IHI) in Cambridge, Massachusetts.

From 1973 until 1983, Dr. Schellekens was a general practitioner in Leiden, The Netherlands. From 1983 till 1989, he was a medical advisor of the Dutch Healthcare Insurance Board (Ziekenfondsraad) in Amstelveen. In 1989, he was appointed as the chief medical officer of the Reinier de Graaf Gasthuis, a 760-bed acute care teaching hospital in Delft.

Since 2000, Dr. Schellekens has been Senior Fellow and international liaison of IHI. He can be reached at w.schellekens@cbo.nl.

Both Dr. Reinertsen and Dr. Schellekens were successful medical doctors (rheumatology and family practice) and subsequently became chief executive officers of major healthcare institutions (Park Nicollet Health Services in Minneapolis; CareGroup in Boston; and Reinier de Graaf Hospital in Delft, The Netherlands). In addition, both are highly visible leaders in the quality improvement movement.

The combined clinical, administrative, and quality

improvement experience of these two physician executives and their connections to the best minds in quality on two continents give them a unique perspective on the current strongest ideas for improvement.

ACKNOWLEDGMENTS

This book would not have come about if there were not a place to generate ideas, to share experience with ideas, and to infect others with the ideas that get results. We are especially grateful to Don Berwick and Maureen Bisognano for creating that place—the Institute for Healthcare Improvement.

The ideas presented in this book have been generated, used, and refined by hundreds of innovators in the world, especially those within the Dutch Institute for Healthcare Improvement CBO and the Institute for Healthcare Improvement. The faculty, staff, and members of these organizations have put these ideas into action and continue to teach us what works and what does not.

We acknowledge the special contributions of Tom Nolan, Andrea Kabcenell, Mary Minniti, Nancy Bitting, Marc Pierson, Kirstie Galbraith, Jacqui Close, Sarah Garrett, Jo Bibby, Göran Henriks, Mats Bojestig, Sven-Olof Karlsson, Ed Wagner, Roger Resar, Carol Haraden, Gene Litvak, Brian Jarman, Duncan Moore, Mark O'Bryant, Winnie Schmeling, Rob Colones, Donna Isgett, Marie Segars, Rick Shannon, Paul O'Neill, David Jackson, Justine Carr, Ralph de la Torre, Darla Belt, Uma Kotagal, John Bucuvalas, Davy Crockett, Bill Rupp, Michael Pugh, Jannes van Everdingen, Caroline van Weert, Marius Buiting, Peter van Splunteren, Teus van Barneveld, Anja Evers, Cecile Frijns, Maike Verhoeven, Marian Tervoort, Jan Koning, Jos Immerzeel, and Elmer Mulder. They all still inspire us with their quest for quality.

Frank Davidoff has made this a far better book than it could ever have been, with his detailed, superb reviews and suggestions for every chapter.

Finally, we are grateful to two individuals—our wives, Cheryl and Marijke. They have put up with our ideas for decades and helped us to sort the wheat from the chaff.